T0168954

COPING
with
HEARING LOSS

Plain Talk for Adults About Losing Your Hearing

COPING
with
HEARING LOSS

Plain Talk for Adults
About Losing Your Hearing

by SUSAN V. REZEN, Ph.D.
and CARL D. HAUSMAN Ph.D.

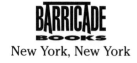

BARRICADE
BOOKS
New York, New York

Published by Barricade Books Inc.
150 Fifth Avenue
Suite 700
New York, NY 10011

Library of Congress Cataloging-in-Publication Data

Rezen, Susan V.
    Coping with hearing loss : a plain talk for adults suf-
fering from hearing loss / Susan V. Rezen and Carl
Hausman.—Rev. ed.
        p.   cm.
    Includes index.
    ISBN: 1-56980-165-7
        1. Presbycusis—popular works. 2. Deafness—
Popular works. I. Hausman, Carl, 1953-   . II. Title.
RF291.5.A35R49   2000
362.4'2—dc20
                                                    92-36728
                                                        CIP

Printed in the United States of America.
10 9 8 7 6 5 4 3 2 1

DEDICATION:
To our spouses, old and new—who put up with us.

Contents

INTRODUCTION

Having a hearing loss means more than just not being able to hear well. It can bring on a wide range of problems that, at first, you might not suspect have any link to your hearing: isolation from family and friends, a feeling of inadequacy in social situations, and a decline in your overall self-image.

Unfortunately, the social and psychological problems that accompany a hearing impairment are not always immediately obvious, and to make matters worse, the people who should be helping you, often do not. Physicians and audiologists (non-medical hearing specialists) sometimes lack the training and inclination to tackle these particular problems, and therefore may brush aside the vocational, social, and emotional aspects. Dealing with the physical problem, you see, is frequently a rather cut and dried affair, but helping a patient cope with hearing loss is not.

The purpose of this book is to help you and your family cope with that hearing loss. It will touch on matters as practical as communicating with a mumbling bank teller, choosing hearing aids, and dealing with doctors. It will also explore some more abstract but equally important concepts: how impaired hearing affects the relationship between husband and wife, why people are reluctant to admit that they don't have perfect hearing,

1

and why they are sometimes just as reluctant to do something about it.

Another section will deal with learning how to adjust to, and use, hearing aids. As you may already have found out, hearing aids simply cannot restore normal hearing, and it takes a certain amount of skill to use them well.

Rehabilitative hearing therapy will also be discussed: what it involves, where it's offered, and how it can turn things around for an unhappy person struggling with the self-imposed isolation of a hearing disability. Information on dealing with tinnitus, ringing or roaring sounds in the ears, is included.

One chapter will explain how the ear functions when it is working correctly, and what happens when it is not. In case this seems as though it will be a bit tedious, remember that a problem rarely seems as frightening or puzzling once you understand what is happening. A basic knowledge of the ear is also helpful when dealing with doctors, audiologists, and hearing aid dispensers.

Medical terms are explained as you read along. In addition, the Glossary at the end of the book will tell you the meaning and pronunciation of these and other terms that may be unfamiliar to you. And the appendix on Internet use with hearing loss can help you expand your knowledge well beyond this book.

It is most important to remember that you are not alone. Hearing loss affects about 28 million Americans; about 25 percent in ages forty-five to sixty-five and about 35-40 percent of people over age sixty-five have a hearing loss.

Throughout, this book will trim away the fat and serve up only the lean—the practical knowledge gathered by helping thousands of people learn to live and listen in spite of their hearing loss. There is only one requirement on your part: You have to want to help yourself. To adjust to hearing aids you must practice an entirely new way of listening, and to cope with reduced hearing you must be willing to change some of your attitudes and behavior. All this can only be accomplished after you admit to yourself that there is a problem and decide to confront it.

But since you picked up this book in the first place—and are still reading it—you're already well on your way.

{ 1 }
Why Am I Losing My Hearing

Ears, unfortunately, are somewhat like automobiles: They can malfunction, can be damaged, and often just wear out.

In some cases, disease or heredity conspire to rob the hearing mechanism of its function. Many of us suffer noise damage to the ears, often from exposure to machinery or firearms. Adults with a hearing impairment often have an age related hearing loss—meaning that as they grew older, their hearing mechanism lost some of its former ability to pick up and transmit sound.

Hearing loss will happen to almost everyone, it just affects some sooner than others. If we all lived to be a hundred and fifty, everyone would have a hearing loss. But hearing loss is not confined to older people. Recent data show that since the 1970's hearing problems among ages 45-64 are up over 25%, and among ages 18-44, are up by almost 20%. At least 15% of children in the 6-19 age range are showing signs of hearing loss.

For most, loss of hearing begins at age fifty-five to sixty–five, but age–related hearing loss can begin as early as the mid thirties, slightly earlier for men than women. Hearing impairment ranks fifth in chronic health conditions among all ages in the United States. Among those over 65, hearing loss ranks third among the most often-reported chronic conditions, following arthritis and hypertension. Hearing loss due to disease or noise damage can occur at any age, but often compounds the problems encountered due to the aging process. Many cases of hearing loss—at least 10 million of the 28 million total cases in the U.S.—are a result of noise damage.

Age–related hearing loss, known scientifically as *presbycusis* (pronounced prez–buh–CUE–sis), is not medically dangerous, nor is it a symptom of senility or any mental problem. Because there is no way for you to be sure that your hearing loss stems from presbycusis, it is important to see a physician, who can diagnose your problem with a painless examination. It is essential that you see a doctor immediately if your hearing loss comes on suddenly, or is accompanied by pain, dizziness, severe ringing or roaring sensations, a feeling of pressure, or drainage from the ear. These symptoms could indicate a medically significant condition, such as a metabolic imbalance, a circulatory problem, or other disease.

As part of your examination, a physician will probably have your hearing evaluated by an *audiologist*, a communication specialist who tests hearing, recommends and fits hearing aids and other hearing-help technologies, and provides counseling and therapy to help clients deal with a hearing disability. Both the physician (either your family doctor or an ear, nose, and throat specialist) and the audiologist will probably use terms that are unfamiliar to you, which is one more reason to arm yourself in advance with some background into the workings of the marvelous mechanism of the ear.

By understanding the ear's function, you will also have a better grasp of what can go wrong with it, and how this situation can be helped. Also, a thorough understanding of what is happening can ease some of the perfectly natural apprehension you feel when something inside you is not working quite right. Let's take a look at the structure of an ear, as shown in Figure 1.

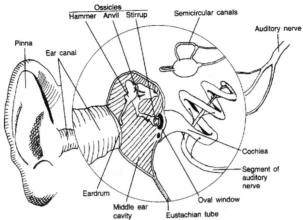

Figure 1.1 The structure of the human ear

The ear is divided into three parts: the outer ear, middle ear, and inner ear. The outer ear consists of the pinna (the structure of skin and cartilage that hangs on the side of your head) and the ear canal, which extends about an inch into the head.

The human pinna serves as a collector of sound, although not a particularly efficient one. Many animals, dogs for example, have movable pinnas that point in the direction of the sound; some members of the fox family have pinnas so large and mobile that they can detect the sound of ants moving underground. The acoustic (sound-shaping) properties of the pinna also enhance certain pitches important for understanding speech and for helping us locate the direction of a sound source.

From the pinna, the sound enters the ear canal, which serves two basic purposes. It protects the fragile eardrum from the elements, and also increases the loudness of certain pitches that are important for understanding speech. These particular pitches are enhanced in the canal by resonance, much the same way in which the sound of your breath is amplified when you blow over the top of a soda bottle.

The middle ear is made up of the eardrum, ossicles,

and the eustachian tube. The eardrum (called a tympa-num in medical terminology) is a delicate, pearly–white membrane stretched tightly over the end of the ear canal. The eardrum is highly sensitive to vibration, and sound is nothing more than a vibration in the air. After the eardrum picks up this vibration, it passes it along to the ossicles, three tiny bones called the hammer (malleus), anvil (incus), and stirrup (stapes). The ossi-cles amplify the intensity of the vibration by taking the movement of the comparatively large eardrum and com-pressing it, so that all the vibration is focused on the minuscule footplate of the stirrup.

This ingenious internal amplifier works best in an air–filled environment which is provided by the eustachian tube. This tube opens on one end in the mid-dle ear, and on the other end in the back of the throat. It allows replacement of air absorbed by tissues in the middle ear, drains off accumulated fluid inside, and pro-vides a way to equalize air pressures inside and outside of the middle ear. The sensation of the tube opening is felt when your ears "pop" as you ride up an elevator or climb a steep hill.

The inner ear consists of the cochlea (the Latin word for snail), the semicircular canals, and the endings of the auditory nerve. The base of the cochlea and the footplate of the stirrup meet at what's called the oval window, a tissue–covered opening that separates the middle and inner ear and transmits vibration. There is another tissue–covered opening called the round win-dow, which equalizes pressure by moving out when the oval window is pressed in to the inner ear by the foot-plate of the stirrup.

The intense vibration of the footplate sets up a wave in the fluid filled cochlea. This wave sets in motion tiny hairlike projections inside the cochlea, which are in contact with the nerve endings. These hair cells, as they are called, translate this motion into nerve impulses, which are carried through the acoustic nerve. This nerve brings the signals to the brain for processing. The semicircular canals do not affect hearing, but they do help you maintain balance by sensing the position of the fluid inside them, giving your body a method to tell if it is level or moving, even if your eyes are closed.

A number of problems can arise within the entire hearing mechanism. One of the most common discomforts is the accumulation of wax (called *cerumen*) in the ear canal. But wax protects the ear from infections and keeps it moist so the ear canal doesn't itch. Thus, some wax is good, and routinely cleaning it out can cause problems. If the ear is plugged with wax, sound cannot travel through it as well. This condition is actually brought on by efforts to clean the inside of the ear, as it pushes the wax farther into the ear canal and impacts it. So don't try and clean out the ear canal; just wash the outside of the ear with a washcloth.

Trying to take out your own wax or wax from a child's ear can lead to a hole in the eardrum or injury to the sensitive skin of the ear canal. Amateur attempts at removing wax can also lead to excess moisture, which can cause fungus or bacterial infections such as "swimmer's ear."

The ear normally has a mechanism to clean itself, although this mechanism can and does malfunction. Impacted cerumen is quite common. In the over fifty-five age group, twenty-five percent of men and nineteen percent of women have this problem. Check with your doctor if you think there is too much wax in your ears. A physician is able to remove wax quickly, safely, and painlessly. Your doctor may suggest that you use an over-the-counter earwax removal product which makes the wax soft and moist so it doesn't impact into a hard barrier to sound. If you use it, get help with putting the liquid in your ears because if you do it yourself, it may just run out again. But beware, in inexperienced hands the use of the syringe to flush the wax out often just pushes the wax further in.

You can also have a problem with too little wax (which can be caused by washing the ears out too frequently). The dry flakey skin which results is very itchy and can lead to abrasions when you scratch—an open invitation for infections. Use of a natural oil like olive or vegetable oil will moisturize the skin, increase water rejection and soften ear wax. Glycerin drops or moisturizing creams also help. Tough cases may require over-the-counter low-level hydrocortisone creams at night. But best bet, if it persists, is to check with your doctor.

Another relatively common problem is a perforated eardrum, that is, a hole in the eardrum, as a result of injury or infection. Such a perforation will probably allow a mucous fluid to drain out of the ear canal, and will allow germs to enter, causing frequent infections.

The space behind the eardrum, the middle ear, is the source of most childhood earaches and infections, but adults can have such problems as well. You know the "plugged" feeling you get in your ears during a cold? Well, the problem is the swelling in your throat, a swelling that restricts the opening of the eustachian tube. When air can't get up the eustachian tube, a slight vacuum is formed in the middle ear. This draws the fluid from the tissues into the middle ear, and the fluid can't drain out because the eustachian tube is blocked. The fluid alone is enough to cause a problem, but if that fluid gets infected you're in for a bout of *otitis media* (middle ear infection or inflammation) that can be annoying and even painful.

There are several other problems that can crop up in the middle ear. One of the three bones, the stirrup, can have a bony growth around it, a condition known as otoclerosis. This growth "cements" the stirrup in place so that the vibrations are not properly passed to the inner ear. This happens more often in women and is made worse by pregnancy. Otosclerosis also tends to run in families, but can skip people or generations.

All of these problems cause what's called a *conductive hearing loss*, the outer or middle ear does not conduct sound as well as it should. The result of a conductive loss is primarily a loss of sensitivity for hearing soft sounds; once sound is loud enough, though, it can be heard adequately.

Now let's move farther into the head. The inner ear is a very fragile organ, and there are several things that can go wrong with it. One of the inner ear's worst enemies is excessive exposure to noise. Noise exposure causes tiny hair cells to be banged around, and the violent waves produced by huge vibrations will eventually cause the hair cells to break. If you already have a hearing loss, it is important to be very careful of noise exposure because a hearing impaired person is often highly susceptible to noise damage. What are some of the clues if you're being over-exposed to noise?

- if you must raise your voice to talk above the noise
- if you have a ringing or roaring sensation after the exposure
- if people seem to mumble after you've been exposed to the noise

You are also more susceptible to noise exposure damage if you are exposed to combinations of certain toxic chemical agents, to some drugs such as those used in chemotherapy, to stress brought about from disliking the noise source, and even from stress caused by physical exercise like aerobics.

Remember that when the situation calls for you to wear hearing protection, such as muffs or commercially-available earplugs, do so. Also, if you must be exposed to noise, take breaks from the noise. The ear tolerates noise much better when there is a break, even a short one, during which it can recuperate. Don't forget, by the way, that there are many potentially damaging noise sources in addition to the usual suspects of chainsaws, guns, and power tools. Keep in mind leaf blowers, motorcycles, subway trains, and even lawnmowers and snowblowers as a potential source of hearing damage.

Noise affects the ear in different ways. Long-term exposure to moderately loud noise over years causes damage to outer hair cells which cause you to lose your ability to hear soft sounds (sensitivity), but extremely loud noise, sometimes even with short exposure, damages inner hair cells which carry the information to the brain. This causes problems in understanding speech even when it is loud enough. (We'll talk more about this in a few pages.) Beware of the attitude that you can tolerate the noise until symptoms occur. By the time you begin having trouble following conversation, you have lost 30% of the hair cells.

Remember that a proper supply of oxygen is crucial for the health of the inner ear. Problems with circulation (high blood pressure, arteriosclerosis, thrombosis, coronary conditions), the kidneys, or the lungs can contribute to a hearing loss. Metabolic imbalances such as thyroid problems and diabetes can affect hearing. A common problem is Meniere disease (also called *endolymphatic hydrops*), where there is too much inner-ear fluid. Meniere disease can cause episodes of fluctuating hearing loss, a feeling of fullness in the ears, severe dizzy spells, and a roaring sound in the ears.

Speaking of diseases, the inner ear is subject to infection by a variety of viruses, which are often blamed for sudden losses where no other cause is evident. These types of viruses are specific to the inner ear, but other ailments affecting the entire body can also cause a hearing loss. Mumps, measles, and influenza for instance, are sometimes responsible; actually, any disease accompanied by an extremely high fever can damage the hearing mechanism.

Tobacco, either from first-hand or second-hand smoke, restricts blood flow and brings about a deficiency of oxygen in the blood, both of which conditions can harm your hearing. A recent study in the *Journal of the American Medical Association* showed that smokers have a 70% greater risk of developing hearing loss in middle or old age than those who don't smoke. The odds increase with the amount of smoking. For every 10 "pack-years" of smoking (packs per day for x number of years) the risk increases by 5% for people less than 70. Tobacco's effects have also been known to impair vision.

Besides nicotine in tobacco, there are other common drugs that can cause hearing loss and/or ringing in the ears. Any medicine with aspirin or quinine in it can cause these symptoms temporarily if taken in large quantities. Some prescription drugs can have these effects, but your physician or pharmacist should tell you about it.

Further along the tract leading from the ear up to the brain, there is the possibility of tumors, but this is a very rare condition and is accompanied by other medical symptoms besides hearing loss.

How does age affect the hearing mechanism? For one thing, many components of the ear deteriorate over the years. The eardrum, for example, can become too thick or too thin. In the cochlea, there may be stiffening as well as some deterioration of the hair cells; nerve pathways may also degenerate somewhat, and the signal from the ear might not be transmitted clearly to the brain.

This lack of clear transmission doesn't always show up on standard hearing tests but results in lengthened reaction time and shortened attention/memory span, and causes trouble in following fast conversation, paying attention to conversation for a long time, switching topics, and picking out what we want to hear in noise or with multiple talkers.

When changes from disease, injury, or age occur in the inner ear, they sometimes bring about what's called "nerve deafness." Unfortunately, this term is quite misleading. Nerve deafness not only has nothing to do with being nervous, but the person is also not completely deaf; the loss may be of any degree of severity. What is called nerve deafness refers to damage or destruction of mechanisms in the cochlea and auditory nerve, causing reduced sensitivity to sounds and difficulty in understanding speech. Doctors call this a *sensorineural hearing loss*. Sensorineural loss has been linked to a variety of psychosocial dysfunctions such as depression, hypertension and stress, and dependent living.

This type of hearing problem, whether we term it nerve deafness or sensorineural hearing loss, can cause decreased capacity in either one or both of two distinct abilities: *sensitivity* to sounds and *discrimination* of sounds.

Sensitivity involves the ability to detect soft sounds. People with a sensitivity loss may not be able to hear a whisper or a bird singing, but once the sound is loud enough for them, they can interpret it correctly. *Discrimination* refers to the ability to clearly distinguish one sound from another; discrimination is the ability that allows understanding of speech. People with a discrimination problem as well as a sensitivity problem will find that even if speech is made loud enough for them to hear, they will still misunderstand what is being said. It is rather like listening to someone with a heavy accent.

Having them talk louder doesn't make it any easier to understand. As another example, turning up a radio with poor reception still doesn't make the sound clear.

Most sensorineural hearing losses involve various combinations of sensitivity and discrimination problems. Sensitivity is measured in decibels, a rather complicated measurement of loudness. Instead of trying to explain the mathematical definition of a decibel, let's look at the decibel measurements of some common sounds to get an idea of what we are talking about. Note that just to make things more complicated, there are different types of decibel measurements, so other scales may not seem to agree. The measure we are using here is the type most commonly used in discussions of hearing loss.

0 decibels	The softest sound a typical ear can hear
20 decibels	A whisper
45 decibels	Soft conversational speech
55 decibels	Loud conversational speech
65 decibels	Loud music from a radio
75 decibels	City traffic
100 decibels	A loud factory
110 decibels	A loud amplified rock band
120 decibels	A chain saw or other loud power tool
140 decibels	A jet engine at takeoff
160 decibels	A gun firing

Now that we're on speaking terms with decibel levels, let's turn this example around and observe how a loss of a certain amount of hearing affects communication. For example, a person with a 50–decibel loss obviously cannot hear sounds that have a loudness of 50 decibels or less, and will therefore find even loud conversational speech extremely soft.

A hearing level of 15 decibels or less is not considered a problem. Proceeding from that point:

Decibel Loss	Hearing Problem
16–25	A slight loss only causes problems if the listening conditions are very poor, as at a noisy party, or if someone speaks very softly, perhaps at a church or library.
26–40	A loss of from 26 to 40 decibels is considered a mild hearing loss. But "mild" can be misleading because losses in this range can cause significant communication problems. Good communication is possible in ideal listening situations, but background noise will make it hard to hear. Also causing difficulty: soft-spoken people, speakers not facing you, and speakers more than 10 feet away. Use of hearing aids (hearing aids will be discussed in Chapter 6) will be helpful.
41–55	Moderate hearing loss. Conversation can be heard at a distance of three to five feet, but understanding speech is usually a strain, especially in background noise. Full-time use of hearing aids is necessary.
56–70	Moderately severe hearing loss. Conversation must be very loud and close by to be heard at all, and very little can be heard in group situations. Hearing aids are needed, but may not be the whole solution at times because clarity is affected even when sound is sufficiently loud. Speechreading instruction (to be dealt with in Chapter 11) and

speech therapy and counseling (to be dealt with in Chapter 12) are helpful.

71–90   Severe hearing loss. Only very loud speech, about one foot away from the ear, can be heard, and it is often quite distorted. (You can simulate this effect by putting your hand tightly over your mouth as you talk.) Hearing aids will provide some benefit, but speechreading training and counseling are also needed. Work with a speech therapist may be needed to keep speech from deteriorating (speech sounds may become distorted when the speaker can not hear himself correctly).

91-120   Profound hearing loss, or deafness. Some extremely loud sounds may be heard (or felt through vibration). Training in speechreading, speech therapy, and counseling are absolutely essential. Use of hearing aids may help with speechreading, but cannot be used primarily to understand speech. Lipreading or sign language is the primary source.

120+   Total deafness. The only sensation is vibration when the sound is extremely loud. Essentially, there is no hearing, just feeling.

Most people lose hearing in both ears, but a significant number—6.5 million—have one-sided, or unilateral, hearing losses. Many people don't realize until later in life that they don't have usable hearing in one ear. Perhaps they put the phone up to the ear they hardly ever use and notice that they cannot hear. Some people are born with a unilateral hearing loss or lose hearing in one ear because of disease or injury.

A unilateral hearing loss makes it much more difficult to localize sound. It increases hearing problems in background noise, especially if the noise comes from the side of the good ear. Another difficulty comes from speakers directly on the bad side. Speech will be audible but sound distorted. But if they are even slightly towards the front or are a few feet away from the bad ear, the good ear should compensate fairly well in good listening conditions. When people report that they don't hear well because of a hearing loss in one ear, they usually have a loss in both ears, but one is worse so the better ear seems normal.

One dilemma caused by sensitivity losses, even mild ones, is that they frequently are most severe at higher pitches, or more correctly, higher frequencies. Many consonants are high–pitched sounds formed by air exploding or hissing from the mouth, such as *f, s, v, sh, th, ch, p, k, z,* and *t*. When the ear can't properly receive these high–frequency sounds, words like "Sue," "chew," and "shoe" may all sound the same, and the context of the sentence must be used to fill in the missing sounds. Even if you can't hear the sh in "I've got a hole in my shoe," you can still figure out what was said by the meaning of the rest of the sentence. However, if you must figure out too many words from context, the task becomes too difficult and the conversation can not be followed. Soon, it becomes difficult to determine if you really can't hear or whether you are just "tuning out."

It is important to reinforce the notion that a high-frequency loss does cause you to "hear but not understand." High pitches are critical for understanding speech, and when they are not perceived the effect is, indeed, like "everyone mumbling." Problems arise especially in background noise.

Unfortunately, people with high-frequency losses may encounter those who accuse them of "having a short attention span," or "hearing only when they want to." Indeed, this may appear to be the case when people observe your behavior in background noise. A high-frequency loss does seem to shorten your attention span when in fact you are actually listening attentively. This occurs because it is difficult and tiring to follow the conversation when you're in background noise. Often, when it is quiet, it appears like you have suddenly decided that you "want to hear."

As you can see, there are many levels of hearing loss, so just telling people that you are "deaf" isn't a good idea. In fact there is a definite difference between being hard of hearing and being deaf. People who are *hard of hearing* still use their hearing as their primary means of communication, assisted by lipreading and technology such as hearing aids. They are usually looking for some kind of cure or remediation for their problem and tend to integrate into the hearing world. They rarely use or need sign language. Those who are *deaf* cannot use their hearing as their primary mode, but may use it to help their lipreading or sign language when communicating with hearing people. There is another category called those who are Deaf (note the captial D). These people are usually profoundly deaf from a very early age, if not birth, who use American sign language and prefer not to use their voice or lipreading. They are proud of being deaf and thus do not want to be "fixed" by hearing aids or surgery because they believe there is nothing "broken". They tend to form their own culture, marrying other deaf, preferring deaf children, and using their own language.

Now let's consider discrimination, and how it affects communication. This ability to distinguish one sound from another is measured by determining what percentage of a list of one–syllable words can be correctly recognized when presented at comfortable loudness (this test will be explained in greater detail in Chapter 8). Identifying individual words is harder than picking them up in a conversation, however, so keep in mind that a discrimination score (also called a word recognition score) of 70 percent means that you can pick up more than seven out of ten words during a conversation because you have the advantage of context.

Ninety-percent discrimination, by the way, is considered the lower limit for normal hearing, meaning that someone at this level will have hardly any problem communicating, assuming that speech is presented loudly enough to eliminate any trouble caused by a loss of sensitivity. When the discrimination ability drops below normal, these problems arise:

Discrimination Ability	Hearing Problem
75–90%	Mild difficulty understanding speech, especially in background noise. The mind is able, though, to fill in the gaps and figure out what was said in most situations. This is similar to talking over the telephone.
60–75%	Moderate difficulty in communication. Speech often seems distorted, and it is difficult to follow a conversation.
45–60%	Moderately severe difficulty communicating. Techniques such as watching lips must be used to fill in the gaps and understand what is being said.

Below 45%   Speech sounds almost like a foreign language, and there is severe difficulty in communication unless the hearing is combined with lipreading.

Just amplifying the loudness of the sound does not necessarily help a discrimination problem, although when there is also a drop in sensitivity, hearing aids can be beneficial. Hearing distorted speech through a hearing aid is better than hearing no speech without an aid.

There is no way for you to accurately test your own hearing, but it's safe that if you think you have a loss, you probably do, and should have your hearing evaluated. If you're not sure about whether you have a hearing problem (remember, it can sneak up over a period of years and is not always obvious to you), try asking yourself a few questions.

- Do I tune out from conversations where there is more than one person talking?
- Am I letting my spouse or my best friend do most of my talking for me?
- After a long conversation, am I usually tired and irritable?
- When I answer people's questions, do they often appear puzzled or embarrassed by my response?
- Does it seem that my friends and family are avoiding conversation with me?
- Do I frequently misunderstand people, and ask them to repeat what they have said?
- Do I hear sound but not understand speech clearly?
- Do I think that people mumble?
- Do I have trouble hearing when there is noise around?
- Do I turn up the TV louder than others do?
- Do I have a "good ear" for the telephone or to turn toward the speaker?

- Do I have trouble hearing when I can't see the speaker's face or I am far away?
- Is there ringing or buzzing in my ears?

If you answered yes to one or more of these questions, it's possible that you have a hearing loss, one that you may not even be conscious of. An evaluation by an audiologist can determine how bad your loss is, whether your particular hearing loss is worse at certain frequencies, and whether it involves sensitivity or discrimination loss (or both).

It's worth mentioning at this point that a closely related problem to hearing loss known as tinnitus (pronounced either TIN–ih–tuss or tin–IGH-tuss) affects about 40 million people in the United States. Tinnitus is usually described as a ringing or roaring sound in the ear or head; some people describe it as like the whistling of the wind or the sound of crickets. While tinnitus often accompanies an age–related hearing loss, the two do not necessarily occur together. We will address tinnitus at length in Chapter 11.

Although this short course in the nature of a hearing loss leaves a lot of ground uncovered, it should have provided you with enough background to understand your hearing loss and discuss it with a doctor or audiologist. There are certainly some questions you would still like answered, so we'll deal with a few of the questions most commonly asked at this point.

How much worse will my hearing loss become?
Unfortunately, there is no way to make an accurate prediction. Recent research has shown that some age related hearing losses stabilize around the age of sixty-five, though there's no guarantee of that happening. If your loss is due to noise exposure, you can prevent further damage by staying out of

the noise, or by using earmuffs or earplugs to reduce the intensity of the noise. Progression of loss due to heredity or disease will vary with the specific cause. The best tactic is to have your hearing tested every two years after your initial visit to a doctor and audiologist. If there is a change, your hearing should be tested more frequently after that.

Why me, and not my friends who are the same age?
Some of them hear very well. Some people are predisposed toward a hearing loss, just as some people are more likely to gain weight, have heart trouble, or develop high blood pressure. Heredity plays a part, so if your parents or siblings developed presbycusis at an early age, you may have inherited a tendency toward it. Exposure to noise, such as years of work in a foundry, can also hasten the effects of an oncoming loss. Your general health, now and through your entire life also plays a role in determining how well your hearing will hold up in later years.

Is it permanent?
Yes, except for a few cases that will respond to medical or surgical treatment (explained in Chapter 7).

I sometimes get the impression I am speaking too loudly or softly. Can that be the case?
Probably. If you have a conductive hearing loss, you probably speak too softly because of the occlusion effect which you can simulate by plugging your ears when you talk. Most people with a sensorineural loss usually speak more loudly than appropriate so that they may hear themselves more clearly. But at times they may also speak too softly, usually in background noise. Since hearing

impaired people don't hear the background noise well or at all, they don't know to raise their voice above it.

The best strategy is to gauge the situation and how people react. If folks you are talking to seem to back away, you can lower your voice. If you're in background noise—heavy traffic out the window or a fan blowing in the room—you may want to raise your level. Others may also comment that your own speech is not sharp and clear, especially on sounds like s, sh, f. This is because you are not hearing them sharply and clearly. Try making an effort to enunciate well.

You talk about going to see a doctor or an audiologist. Which one should I see first?

It really doesn't matter, since you will probably have to see both. A doctor will refer you to an audiologist, and if the doctor you see is an ear, nose, and throat specialist, an audiologist may be there on the staff. An audiologist will probably want you to see a doctor to make sure there is no medical problem.

What about telephone hearing tests? Couldn't they substitute for a visit to a doctor or an audiologist?

While telephone hearing tests have become common, we're rather skeptical about their reliability. However, they do raise awareness of hearing problems.

My doctor told me that I have a 60% hearing loss. Does that mean I have a 60 db loss or I hear 60% of what is said?

Physicians often give a percentage because they think we will have trouble understanding decibels. But expressing the level of hearing loss by percentage can be misleading. (In fact, sometimes physicians just give the decibel level as a percentage, which is not valid.) A true percentage involves a mathematical formula developed by the American Medical Association for use in legal cases. But that formula does not consider some of the high pitches which are important for understanding speech and it considers someone with a slight loss to have no problems. Also, a 100% loss does not mean total deafness. Thus, someone with a 2% loss or even 0% loss can be a candidate for hearing aids. Ask for a description of your loss in terms such as mild, severe, and so forth, and how your loss will affect communication.

The audiologist said my hearing was normal for my age. Why do I still have problems hearing?

A lot of things are normal for people as they get older—high blood pressure, fading eyesight, and arthritis. But this does not mean we should avoid getting help! Yes, it's normal to lose some hearing with age, but that will cause difficulty in many aspects of your life. And you can be helped.

Can you protect or improve your hearing with your diet?

A nutritious diet helps your general health including the function of your heart, lungs, and kidneys— all of which are important for getting oxygen and nutrients to your ears. A high fat diet may raise your cholesterol and decrease blood flow. In fact, a few studies have shown a slight improvement in hearing with a lowering of cholesterol. Hearing loss has also been associated with low amounts of vitamin B-12 and folic acid in the blood. However, there is still no hard evidence as to what is the best "ear food."

Doesn't the future hold some cures for hearing loss?

The improvement of the cochlear implant is already in progress (see the chapter on hearing aids), but will not be used for less-than-severe losses for a long time. There is work in much earlier stages on hair cell regeneration and gene therapy. But those are many years from realization. The theory that noise induced hearing loss may be due to overtaxed hair cells emitting increasing amounts of free radical molecules that cause the damage, may someday lead to anti-oxidant therapy.

{ 2 }
The Psychological Effects of Hearing Loss

Millions of people go through needless emotional suffering simply because they have not been adequately prepared to cope with their hearing disability. Professionals in the hearing field, who may be experts at treating the physical side of a hearing loss, often don't have the time or motivation to explain and help deal with a client's typical anxieties and emotions.

In the case of an age–related hearing disability, for example, the psychological effects that go hand in hand with the physical problem are just as much a natural part of the aging process as the hearing loss itself. When these emotional reactions are not dealt with properly they can be magnified all out of proportion, and may even cause drastic personality and lifestyle changes.

Each of us reacts differently to events in our lives, but psychologists have found that almost everyone who endures an emotional or physical loss goes through the same stages of *denial, projection, anger, depression, and acceptance.* Everyone has a right to be angry, to cry, or to feel upset at the world as they go through these stages. Let's examine the impact of these emotional stages on someone who is trying to adjust to a hearing loss.

Denial is a natural initial reaction if you are faced with a threat to your physical or emotional well–being, because it is painful to accept at first, and your emotions seek a way to stall for time to muster the resources to accept this unpleasant fact. At first, it's easy to deny a hearing loss, because it may build up so gradually that it is not perceptible. The denial stage, though, can be—and often is—carried to extremes. A wife, for example may point out to her husband that during the party they just left he didn't catch most of the conversation. "Nonsense," he replies. "I just didn't want to listen to that old windbag." An attitude like this will eventually lead to friction between husband and wife, or among family members. Eventually, though, even the most stubborn person must realize that there is a problem, one that will not go away because it is ignored. Still the mind may not be ready to accept a permanent hearing loss, and will confront the situation bit by bit.

Projection is the next emotional safety valve after denial, and involves blaming your problem on someone else. "Speak up! Why the hell do you mumble all the time?" Remember, though, that there may frequently be some other basis for projection, in addition to your need for a defense mechanism. A commonly heard type of projection is the complaint that "young people nowadays mumble terribly." Well, to a certain extent this is true; without question, there is less attention paid to elocution by our modern school system. However, a person with normal hearing would not have as much trouble understanding a mumbling teenager as would someone with a hearing loss, so it is not logical to conclude that your entire problem in understanding people stems from the way they talk.

Anger usually follows projection, and may take two forms: a generalized "mad at the world" resentment, and a specific anger directed toward an individual, usually the one with whom the hearing impaired person spends the most time. An attitude of continual anger will strain even the strongest relationship, but once again we have to bear in mind that anger in this case may have some basis in reality. A spouse or family member must be careful not to go overboard in pointing out the social blunders of a hearing impaired person, because that type of continual criticism will just bring about more anger. (Chapter 5 will specifically address this problem.)

Depression comes after all anger is vented, and can often be accompanied by acute embarrassment over past behavior, along with isolation and a personality change. An abrupt personality change may leave friends and family rather frightened of the "new person" in their midst, thus heightening the feeling of isolation felt by the hearing impaired person.

Again, remember that there is a *very real* reason for this depression, and one aspect of the cause usually is not even considered by family and friends: There is often a "dead feeling" that comes from not hearing background noise, the sounds that those with good hearing take for granted. Someone with even a mild hearing loss may be saddened consciously or unconsciously, by the fact that birds no longer chirp, downtown no longer hums, and the wind has stopped whistling through the trees.

We also rely on hearing to warn us of impending threats, such as someone approaching from behind, or tampering with the back door. It is quite natural for these feelings of insecurity to aggravate a general depression, and encourage withdrawal and suspicion.

Although this typical depression is understandable, it is far from desirable, and while it probably will happen, at least briefly, to everyone who experiences hearing loss, in some people this emotional stage can linger for years, becoming a virtual life sentence of isolation. Only after chronic depression is seen for what it is—self-imposed exile from the human race—can it be conquered.

Several recent research studies have found that untreated hearing loss has serious emotional and social consequences, especially for older persons. They are more likely to report depression, anxiety and paranoia, and less likely to participate in organized social activities. They feel that other people get angry at them for no reason. Most of the time treatment of the hearing loss results in significant improvement in relationships, in their sense of independence, and even in their social and sex lives.

Acceptance comes after the depression has lifted, and involves the realization that "there is something wrong with my hearing, not with me." This is the only stage where the problems of hearing loss can really be dealt with effectively.

How long does it take to get to the acceptance stage? It's hard to say. For some it may be a matter of days or weeks, while others may need years. But for most it seems to be a matter of months before the realization of a hearing loss can be digested, so to speak. It is important to bear in mind that until you have completely accepted your hearing loss, getting a hearing aid may be futile, or even counterproductive. Your acceptance, or lack of it, is influenced by how you feel about yourself, about others, about the world in general, and how those close to you react to the problem.

Note that there are many other emotions that people report along the path just described. Impatience with those around you causing you to be grouchy at times and then guilty for being so; embarrassment when you realize how you acted during denial, projection, and anger; frustration and ready to give up because you are so tired of struggling to hear.

You probably have noticed that up until this point hearing aids have been mentioned only in passing, and won't be completely covered until Chapter 6. The reason for this is to avoid giving you the impression that getting hearing aids is the only factor in coping with a hearing loss.

Although they are very important and will improve not only your hearing but also your self-image, hearing aids are not a cure-all, nor will they restore all of your lost hearing. Using the aids properly will require diligent practice for the first few weeks of their use. It is essential that a hearing aid user be emotionally ready to cope with the hearing loss and with the difficulties of using the aids. Simply getting hearing aids will not solve your problems.

Many of you wear hearing aids at this point, and are reading this book because you want information on how to use the aids properly. If you have adjusted to your hearing impairment and accepted the fact that you must work to cope with it, the material on better listening habits will benefit you greatly.

Some of you have worn hearing aids in the past, but have since stuck them in the dresser drawer because you were sorely disappointed in their performance (and you probably never received proper instruction and counseling in their use, either). An examination of your emotions at the time you stopped using your aids will probably be very helpful to you.

Most of the readers of this book picked it up in the first place because of an interest in getting first hearing aids, or other, better-suited ones. If you fall into this category, you would be wise to take inventory of your feelings and be sure that you are completely prepared to admit that you need hearing aids and are prepared to learn how to use them. Otherwise, an initial bad experience may rob you of motivation that might never be recaptured.

What might be holding you back? It's possible that you still attach a stigma to wearing hearing aids. Even though people will wear eyeglasses to correct a slight deviation of their vision, they often will resist wearing hearing aids, although they may need them badly.

Perhaps this relates to the fact that many young people wear glasses, and therefore glasses are not viewed as a sign of an age–related disability. Neither should hearing aids.

Maybe you are not yet emotionally ready. It takes time to adjust, certainly, but some people linger in the same stage (usually depression) for years. This usually happens because they did not comprehend what was happening to them emotionally when they were passing through the typical stages following a hearing loss, and therefore *could not cope with feelings that they did not understand.*

Remember that most of what you face in the decision about getting hearing aids is a matter of personal choice. In the past when hearing aids had not been developed or advanced technology was not available, people suffered. But today suffering with a hearing loss is your choice. Going to a professional for help may seem like giving up in your struggle to handle the problem. You are only giving up some of the suffering. And your unwillingness to help yourself is often seen as selfish because of the negative effect on those around you.

It all boils down to learning from the experience of others. Millions of people have been through the same situation you are now facing, and most make it through successfully—but not without their share of mistakes, self-doubt and anxiety. Imagine how much easier it would have been had they been prepared for the emotional difficulties they would encounter along the way! They could have been spared many of the deep-seated suspicions that typically come along in such cases— suspicions that they were becoming senile, or seriously ill, or emotionally disturbed.

Another way to look at the issue of hearing loss is to evaluate the situation using what psychologists and audiologists call "Trychin's concepts," named after a researcher who studied the emotional effects of hearing loss.

These concepts basically involve an analysis of costs versus benefits, and are based on the fact that you actually must *decide* what to do when coping with a hearing loss. *Decide* what will benefit you in the short or long term, how it will benefit you, and what will provide the maximum benefit.

Example: Avoiding social situations.

This provides a short-term benefit because less effort is required on your part. After all, you don't have to go somewhere and expend energy trying to follow conversations, and your personal comfort is increased. But in the long term, this strategy will result in isolation from friends and family.

Example: Getting angry when you can't hear, demanding that others speak up, or blaming the situation on "mumbling."

Again, this provides a short-term benefit. You've vented your frustration and temporarily eased your anger about the hearing problem by blaming it on someone else. But in the long run you'll probably alienate people and isolate yourself more severely than any hearing loss could.

While easier said than done, weighing the benefits and drawbacks of behavior can help you consciously decide how to handle the situation. Perhaps you'll even develop a sense of humor about it, as in the case of one woman we know who wears a large button reading, "Hard of Hearing and Nearsighted—Flirt Aggressively."

No one is maintaining that this is simple, but you can manage the psychological distress of a hearing loss. Here are some basic suggestions.

1. Try to manage the environment. Better lighting, moving chairs to where you can see people's lips, eating at quiet restaurants, are all examples of the kinds of changes you can make by practicing assertive communication behavior. This is covered in some depth in Chapter 13.

2. Manage physical tension. We mentioned biofeedback; that's just one option available to you. Regular physical exercise is also a great way to work off stress.

3. Manage what you think. Your reactions to a situation, not necessarily the situation itself, are what make something stressful. If you view every situation as a disaster, something that is going to cause you immeasurable difficulty, you are probably inventing a self-fulfilling prophecy. But if you believe that coping with a hearing loss is not the worst thing in the world that can happen to you, that it can be managed, that your reactions are what make life stressful, then at least some of the emotional problem can be alleviated.

Our next topic will be an examination of just how these emotional stages affect relationships among family members. First, there are some commonly asked questions concerning the psychological effects of hearing loss that you still may wish answered.

Those emotional stages are interesting, but how can I tell which one I'm in?

It's not all that simple, because these phases are general guidelines and not specific milestones in your psychological process. However, you can get a reasonable idea of where you stand by observing what you do and say when your hearing impairment causes a problem. Here are some typical actions and statements that indicate various stages:

Denial

- Pretending that you heard what was said, giving an inappropriate answer, and then ignoring the fact that your answer didn't make sense to the person with whom you are speaking.
- Claiming a lack of interest or attention when that's really not the case. "I can hear when I want to listen."
- "I'm too young to need hearing aids."
- "I know I don't hear perfectly, but I'm not that bad yet."
- "There's a lot I don't want to hear out there."

Projection

- "The acoustics of this room are lousy."
- "Why can't my nephew learn to stop mumbling?"
- "They don't teach kids how to speak in school today."
- "If my wife really cared about me, she would speak up."

Anger

- "If you're ashamed to be seen with me, why don't you go by yourself?"
- "I hate those Smiths! We had a terrible time at dinner last night, and I won't go out with them again."
- "I'm a good person; what did I ever do to deserve this?"
- "I don't give a damn what the grandchildren say anyway."

Depression

- "I've been making a fool out of myself in front of the Smiths because of this stupid hearing problem, and I'll never be able to face them again."
- "Everything seems so dead, I might as well be dead, too."

• "If I can't do things like I used to, I don't belong in this world any longer."
• "I just have no interest in anything that happens in my family or community any more."

Acceptance
• "I don't want to miss out on things anymore."
• "Even if I can't hear very well, I can still see well and think, and my health is still good."
• "I know it will help out my family if I wear these hearing aids."

How do I know if I have been in a particular stage too long?
It has been too long if the characteristics of a particular stage are harming your lifestyle, personality, or relationships with other people. In other words, you know you're not making much progress when your emotions control you, instead of the other way around.

What should I do if I am not making progress?
Seek professional help, ideally an audiologist with experience in dealing with the social and psychological effects of hearing loss. If you feel capable of it, you can try and work out your own problems, which may be easier now that you have some insight into the nature of a hearing loss and the range of its effects.

I feel that I have pretty well accepted my problem, and want to get it taken care of eventually. Is there any rush?
Yes. Quite often, people reach the acceptance stage but don't take action, and as a result may slip back into other, less productive attitudes. If you feel ready, you should do it now, and the step-by-step course of action you should take will be outlined later in this book.

If the effect of a hearing loss is psychological, why am I so tired?

Trying to communicate when you have a hearing loss is hard work. Tension, frustration, and anxiety do make you physically tired.

My hearing loss seemed to become a major problem right after I retired. Why?

Retirement can be very traumatic. In effect, it's like being told you suddenly can't do the things you were capable of before reaching retirement age. A hearing loss can be a constant reminder that you're "not what you used to be." It's no wonder that the hearing loss seems worse when coupled with an unwelcome retirement.

Retirement also means that you will be spending more time with your spouse, family, or close friends, and your hearing loss affects them, also. The next chapter will explain why you and your family must be aware of your feelings to insure that actions are not misinterpreted, causing a strain on relationships.

Are there any groups that can help?

Yes. A number of organizations offer materials, advice, and guidance as to where to find local support groups. Try:

Self Help for Hard of Hearing People Inc. (SHHH)
7910 Woodmont Ave. Suite1200,
Bethesda MD 20814-3015
 301 657 2248 voice; TTY 301 657 2249
Fax: 301 913 9413
e-mail: national@shhh
Web: www.shhh.org

The National Association for the Deaf
814 Thayer Ave.

Silver Spring, MD 20910-4500
301-587-1788 voice; TTY 301-587-1789
Web: www.nad.org

Association of Late–Deafened Adults
P.O. Box 641763
Chicago, IL 60644
Web: www.alda.org

Better Hearing Institute
515 King Street Suite 420, Alexandria VA 22314
1-800-EAR-WELL
Email: mail@betterhearing.org
Web: www.betterhearing.org

American Speech Language Hearing Association
(ASHA)
10801 Rockville Pike, Rockville MD 20852
Helpline (Toll Free) 1-800-498-2071
www.asha.org

American Academy of Audiology,
8300 Greensboro Drive Suite 750, McLean VA 22102
800 AAA 2336
Fax 703-790-8631
Web: www.audiology.org

{ 3 }
How Hearing Loss Can Ruin a Relationship

We don't always have the power to see ourselves as we really are. Counselors are aware of how difficult it is for some clients to describe a situation in which they are directly involved. To overcome this difficulty, case histories are often presented, because most people find it easier to recognize their behavior when seen in the actions of others.

It is valuable to recognize certain behaviors, especially the ones you want to change. You can't change something until you know what you're dealing with. These case histories of actual relationships affected by hearing loss may throw some light on the matter. See if you recognize yourself.

Case History 1

Depression and Withdrawal. Sally was tolerant. She withstood the blaming and anger of her husband, Arthur, from the onset of his hearing loss. "He's changed," Sally said, "but he's still my husband, and I have to learn to live with this."

When Arthur reached the depression stage, he felt terribly guilty about his treatment of Sally. He began to hate himself for it, feeling that he didn't deserve such a tolerant woman. "She would be better off without me," Arthur felt, and he eventually withdrew into a shell, removing himself from her life.

Sally was bewildered. She couldn't imagine what she had done to make Arthur dislike her (which is how it appeared to her). As a result, she also became depressed and withdrawn.

Case History 2

The Tower of Strength. Frank, a policeman, had always been a powerful and dominant figure in his family; Bea, his wife, and their two children depended on him heavily. But when Frank began to struggle through the typical problems that come with hearing loss, Bea and the children became terrified, because their tower of strength was beginning to crumble. "He's always been so self-confident and capable," she thought, "but he's changed. Where does this leave us?"

Bea began to spend more time with relatives and friends, looking for comfort, as well as someone else to depend on. The boys spent more and more time away from home. Frank, meanwhile, felt deserted. Just when he really needed help from his family, they weren't there.

Case History 3

Continual Confrontation. Evelyn had a hearing loss, and she was mad at the world. Because she was angry almost all the time, life at home was not too pleasant, which made husband Joe angry, too.

Joe began to nag. "You didn't hear a word they said at that party. You made me feel like a fool."

Joe's attitude only made Evelyn angrier. The two fought, literally, every moment they spent together. Because of this situation, Evelyn never did anything about her problem. Why? Because she was angry at Joe, and knew in her own odd way that her hearing problem was the best way to "get back at him," by making him miserable, too.

Case History 4

Passive Aggression. Vivian was mad at the world, too. But she is a quiet woman who wouldn't dream of "making a scene" about the hearing loss of her husband, Cliff.

She spoke very softly, even though Cliff was hardly ever able to hear her the first time. In many cases she would speak with her head turned, and Cliff would become extremely frustrated because he just couldn't understand what was being said.

Vivian is not an aggressive complainer, but she found a quiet and diabolically effective way to take out her long standing anger on Cliff.

Case History 5

Drifting Apart. Agnes and Randall always thought of themselves as the perfect couple, and in many ways they were. The two had survived thirty years of marriage with few quarrels, and it seemed as though they would sail on smooth waters forever.

But when Randall began to experience the emotional problems that accompany hearing loss, he found himself unable to express his feelings to Agnes. "I just can't talk about things like that," he had always felt.

Unlike other couples, they didn't bicker. They didn't place blame. They just began to live separate lives under one roof. Randall felt somewhat ashamed of his "weakness," and Agnes began to feel the same way, too. While they never showed any outward signs of conflict, they had stopped communicating, and neither was very happy.

Case History 6

Suffocating with Kindness. Ellie always thought of herself as the strong one in her marriage with Alfred.

She had always handled all the problems, so why shouldn't she rise to the challenge of Alfred's hearing loss?

Unfortunately, Ellie's idea of help was to take over Alfred's life, and the hearing problem (which Ellie didn't like to talk about) just made things worse. When Alfred, in a period of projection, would say, "The people at that meeting mumbled so badly I couldn't catch a word," Ellie would agree with him, even though she knew it wasn't true.

She thought she was protecting her husband, and acted with the best of intentions, but she was really suffocating him. Even though Alfred might want to go to a party, she would avoid it. "You know you won't like it, Al, so let's just stay home." Still, she would never admit that her husband's problems stemmed from a hearing loss. In effect, she put Alfred in a position where he could not face up to his hearing problem—he couldn't even admit to having one, because his strong–willed wife denied it.

Alfred stayed quiet, but resentful, unable to come to grips with his hearing loss.

Case History 7

Confronting Mortality. Paul, a widower, really enjoyed visits from his son and grandchildren. Lately, though, those visits had been few and far between.

Paul's hearing loss really didn't bother him that much; but his forty-year-old son, Paul Junior, just couldn't cope with it.

Paul Junior just could not handle the fact that his father was getting older. "Dad just isn't the same. He's not himself. I can't stand to see him this way."

True, Paul Senior had his problems. But, at first he regarded his hearing loss as a natural part of the aging process, and nothing to be afraid or ashamed of. So why didn't his son feel the same way?

Paul Junior wasn't really reacting to his father's hearing loss. He was upset because his father was getting older and wouldn't be around forever. (And this also brought home the point that Paul Junior was getting older, too.) Father had always been a stable pillar in young Paul's life, and the hearing loss seemed to point up the fact that no one lives forever.

But Father didn't understand all this. He thought his son was snubbing him because of his hearing problem. Paul Senior became increasingly hurt, angry, and depressed.

Case History 8

Patronizing a Parent. Hal, a successful junior executive, decided that his mother, Clara, was getting senile. "She can hardly carry on a conversation," Hal said. "I've got to start taking care of her. After all, she took care of me for years."

Clara, in the beginning, really didn't feel disabled. She did have some trouble communicating, even with her hearing aid, but did her best to cope.

When Hal began to take over her life, though, her self-image began to change. "Well, maybe there is something wrong with me, or Hal wouldn't act like this."

Eventually, Clara let herself be molded into the role of a weak, dependent old woman—even though she hated it and resented Hal for forcing the role on her.

* * *

You probably have noticed that all the people in these case histories experienced problems because they (or someone close to them) were mired in a stage of denial, projection, anger, or depression. If these psychological stages seemed a bit abstract when they were explained in the previous chapter, perhaps they struck home in the case histories—which is exactly why they were presented.

Before moving on, let's review some of the more common questions about the effects of a hearing loss on a relationship.

I don't seem to fit completely into any of those case histories, but I do recognize myself in bits and pieces of several. Is this normal?

Of course. Not every situation can be pigeonholed into a particular category, and situations are also affected by the personalities of individuals, as well as the condition of the relationship before the hearing loss. Perhaps some people would find that none of the case histories applied.

If the brief descriptions were illuminating, try writing down a similar paragraph or two describing your particular situation. At the risk of being repetitious, we remind you: You can not change something until you know what it is you want to change.

In the example of Clara and her son, you mentioned that her son thought she was senile. What exactly is senility?

It is the physical deterioration of nerve and brain tissue, which is sometimes complicated by inadequate circulation to these tissues. This condition causes problems in memory and abstract thinking. Clara certainly wasn't senile. She just had problems communicating.

Is senility less common than laymen believe?

Yes. Often, problems in communication brought on by hearing loss are mistaken for senility, especially by people who bandy the word about, without really knowing what it means. In some cases, what seems to be senility has been induced by the assortment of drugs sometimes given to older people.

My situation seems so bad that I don't see how it can ever be improved. What can I do?

Things may not be as bad as they seem, but to be

perfectly honest, relationships sometimes do deteriorate to the point where they are irreconcilable. If, after reading the next chapter, you still don't see a light at the end of the tunnel, it is advisable to seek professional help, such as a psychologist, marriage and family therapist, or an audiologist. (Be sure to determine, as best you can, that your psychologist or therapist is interested in and has some knowledge of hearing loss; conversely, if you visit an audiologist be sure that he or she is concerned with rehabilitative counseling. Where to find professional help, and how to choose a therapist, are outlined in Chapters 8 and 12.)

{ 4 }
If You Have a Hearing Loss

To risk oversimplifying the situation, let's consider two short statements that can often get directly to the root of problems associated with hearing loss. **It is not *your* hearing loss; it is *our* hearing loss. It has an effect on everyone around you. It changes your behavior, and therefore alters the way people react to you.**

That sounds pretty simple, doesn't it? Yet these points are often ignored, much to the sorrow of many hearing impaired people who can't understand why things and people have changed.

Even though things change after a hearing loss, your life doesn't necessarily have to change for the worse. You must be willing to accept the facts that you have a permanent hearing loss and that it *will* affect your life and relationships with others, but the loss does not have to harm those relationships. If you can learn from the mistakes of others, there's a very good chance that you can avoid stepping in the same emotional quicksand.

The case histories discussed in the previous chapter were presented with this in mind. Unfortunately, there's no way to say, "in Case History 1, Arthur could have solved all his problems by..." because human relationships are just too complicated for any pat answers.

However, as we've pointed out, once you've identified what is happening to you, it is far easier to deal with; you can use your newly acquired knowledge to develop a healthy attitude about hearing loss and how it may affect your relationships with others. It is also important for you to instill this healthy attitude into those close to you, to insure that they don't sabotage your efforts by clinging to their own reactions of anger, frustration and resentment. It is possible that there will be perceptions of you as unsocial, preoccupied with health matters, forgetful or paranoid. In the early stages of hearing loss, most people are focused on their own problem and don't see the effects on the hearing persons around them.

Just what constitutes a healthy attitude? There are plenty of theories (none of them necessarily correct in every case), but these suggestions have proven useful to most people confronted with a hearing loss.

• Be aware that your hearing loss affects other people, and be prepared to deal with their reactions.

• Find out as much as you possibly can about hearing loss, both in terms of physical and psychological effects. Learn about ways to help yourself communicate more effectively.

• Recognize emotional factors in yourself. Be willing and able to say, "I'm taking out my anger on my wife because she's the only person who will put up with it" or "I accused my husband of mumbling, but it's really my problem, not his."

• Don't become a recluse. People need other people. There are times when you must ask others for help. It's okay to ask for it, but within limits. Don't expect a constant interpreter.

• If you wear hearing aids, don't turn them off as a way to shut out your family and friends or to avoid unpleasant discussions. You owe it to others to be sure your hearing aids are working at their top potential.

• You must be willing to make an honest effort to cope with these problems.

• Admit your problem to those around you, and be prepared to discuss it with people who are affected. You must also fully accept the fact that you do have a problem, but also realize that something can be done to help you deal with it.

• Most people are willing and able to help you communicate better, and you should be willing to accept their assistance. But never forget that dealing with hearing loss is your responsibility. You cannot expect other people to solve your problems, nor should you take out your frustrations on them.

The ultimate goal of coping with a hearing loss is, of course, to feel better about yourself; when that happens, you will improve relations with those around you. Consider, too, that the natural reaction of friends and family who see you taking positive action will be favorable—and they will express this attitude by wanting to help you improve even more.

Let's discuss how this positive attitude could help the people we met in Chapter 3:

The *depression* and *withdrawal* symptoms faced by tolerant Sally and her angry husband, Arthur, probably stemmed from an initial lack of communication. Sally never really understood that her husband was angry about *his hearing loss*, and not angry at *her*. When Arthur became depressed and withdrew, Sally had no way of knowing that his reaction wasn't an expression of dislike for her.

If Arthur had been aware that his hearing loss would affect Sally, and made an effort to deal with her reaction, conditions almost certainly would have been better for both of them.

When strong ex-cop Frank was no longer a tower of strength to his wife, she didn't display a healthy attitude (which is important even though it was not her hearing loss). Bea made no effort to learn about hearing loss, nor to understand that it is not a weakness. Frank didn't help matters much, either; he didn't go out of his way to discuss the problem, or admit that he needed support from his wife (because he thought it would be a sign of weakness).

Both could have coped better if they had recognized their own emotions, owning up to the fact that they were frightened of the "weakness" that they associated with Frank's hearing impairment.

Evelyn and Joe, the unfortunate couple locked in *continual confrontation*, had an unhealthy attitude from the word go. Evelyn should have stopped to consider that her constant anger would have an effect on her husband, making him angry, too; by analyzing her feelings and taking responsibility for her hearing problem, she might have avoided her tragic sin of taking out her anger on someone who cared for her.

Vivian, the specialist in *passive aggression*, made life miserable for her hearing impaired husband. Because of her attitude, any effort by Cliff to help himself would probably be undermined.

How could a healthy attitude have helped? Remember that there's no quick solution in a case such as this (because this relationship might have been in pretty bad shape even before the hearing loss) but bringing the problem out into the open might be a start. By recognizing emotional factors like Vivian's passive aggression, (which may be largely subconscious) the couple would take the first step toward improving their lot, and easing the continual tension between them.

Agnes and Randall, the "perfect couple" who are *drifting apart*, need a better understanding of the nature of a hearing loss and how it is changing their lives.

Alfred, whose wife, Ellie, is *suffocating him with kindness*, has a problem accepting responsibility for his hearing loss. While the problem is shared by both of them, it's up to Alfred to declare that he is a whole person who does not want to be trapped in the role of a social invalid.

Would a better attitude have helped ease the parent/child conflicts described in Chapter 3? If Paul Junior, the son troubled by confronting *mortality* and by his father's aging, could understand the nature of a hearing loss he might be able to tolerate it better. If father Paul knew more about the effects of his hearing loss on his son, Paul would realize that his son is not stopping by as often because of misconceptions and misunderstandings about the hearing impairment (that it indicates frailty or mental derangement). Paul would know that his son still likes him; think how much anguish could be saved by this simple understanding.

Clara, the woman *patronized* by her son Hal, is becoming rapidly convinced that she is a disabled old woman. It's important for Clara to take responsibility for herself, and eliminate debilitating self-doubts. She must convince her well meaning son that the behavior associated with hearing loss does not indicate incompetence or senility.

Don't forget that bringing about an actual change in behavior is a difficult process—much more complicated than the one or two sentence descriptions of what could be accomplished with a healthy attitude. Admittedly, the examples discussed are simplified almost to the point of absurdity; they are presented as illustrations, not step-by-step formulas for personal happiness. There are no such formulas—but the case histories should give you some ideas on how to analyze and confront problems related to your hearing loss.

Experience is an excellent teacher; unfortunately, many of us learn the hard way. The people in the case histories found that dealing with the emotional and social consequences of impaired hearing is actually tougher than facing up to the actual communication problems. That's why so much of this book deals with these complex emotions, in hopes that you can benefit from what others have been through.

Notice that many of the most unhappy people you know suffer from deep-seated resentment of others, of circumstances, or of their own emotional or medical problems. To be frank, the proverbial "chip on the shoulder" is common among people with poor hearing. Blaming others is convenient for them. It is an easy habit to fall into, but it is always a trap. As we've seen, when you take resentment out on others, *they resent you*, and a vicious cycle is formed.

Remember that it is important to stay involved and keep socially active if you want to minimize the negative effects of hearing loss. It is too easy to gradually isolate you and your spouse. When facing going out, there is probably a sense of obligation to family and friends—wanting to see them, but also anxiety at being thrust into a stressful environment.

You probably are thinking that "people go to a party or dinner to wind down and socialize and not to have a ponderous exchange where they have to repeat themselves. It is not relaxing to have to yell responses. It is not fun to be with someone who must strain painfully to understand. And soon, for some people, the burden will be too much and they will look distractedly over my shoulder for someone to rescue them." If this is your line of thinking, you will soon end up hibernating in a safe corner where you fake understanding, smile out of sync, and laugh a step behind the others.

There is an immediate relief of pressure by doing

this, or just not going out at all. *But in the long run it has negative effects.* If your anxiety takes over and keeps you hanging back, others may see you as unapproachable or too vulnerable. However, if others see you at ease, and letting people know how they can interact well with you, little by little you can convince people that you welcome interaction and with a bit of practice, they can enjoy it too.

Here are some of the more common questions asked about the topics covered in this chapter:

If I learn to cope with my hearing loss, can I return to a completely normal life?

No matter how well you cope, or how well you adapt to hearing aids, there are going to be some occupations and activities you just won't be able to handle. However, a hearing loss doesn't have to cripple your lifestyle, and while your life may not be exactly as it always was, it need not be any less worthwhile and rewarding.

I've asked my wife to speak up hundreds of times, but she always forgets. Why?

Old habits die hard. You are asking someone to change a way of speaking she's used for years — all her life, in fact. So be patient. You must provide a lot of feedback, and keep at it. This advice is even more appropriate for those you see less often. They get less practice in changing an established way of speaking. So be willing to put as much effort into your reminders as you expect them to put into a new habit.

How long will it take to make things better?

There's no simple answer to that, other than to warn against expecting overnight results.

As far as being able to cope with just the physical aspects, you'll remember that if you don't currently have hearing aids, you can't expect miracles. If you do have hearing aids, you probably realize by now that it takes effort and practice.

Where emotions are concerned, remember that new behavior has to be practiced until it becomes a habit (taking the place of past behavior, which was also a habit). Think of people you know who have gone on crash diets, only to gain all that weight back. They failed because they didn't make their new behavior (cutting down food intake and increasing activity) a habit. The same theory applies to coping with a hearing loss: You can't just practice a new kind of behavior once or twice and expect it to become part of your lifestyle.

If you can master that new behavior, you're well on your way to establishing a new outlook, which will benefit you and those close to you. Because the people in your life play such a large part in the way you handle a hearing loss, they should read the next chapter, which is specifically written for them.

My husband doesn't want to make love since his hearing has gotten worse. Can a hearing loss affect sexuality?
No, it does not affect your physical sexuality, but it can change your sexual attitude and behavior. Hearing loss often results in feelings of inadequacy and confusion when trying to communicate. This leads to low self–esteem and self-worth. These feelings show up in the bedroom. The person may not feel sexy anymore and/or the spontaneity of passion is frequently lost. Often the person is reluctant to initiate intimate conversations due to the effort involved or for fear of discouraging or frustrating the other person. However, the solution is to

engage in effective communication beforehand.

It is important that the hearing impaired person know that they are still loved and still desired. You must also work out a plan for passionate moments. Do you remove the hearing aids? How do we schedule the romantic moments? Do we keep the lights on for lipreading? How can we have the post lovemaking intimate conversations?

Being successful in a loving relationship means revealing yourself emotionally and becoming vulnerable. That includes demonstrating caring, giving, and commitment as well as the sexual aspect. If the first three are present, communication should be able to work out the last.

Why not try to rejuvenate a stressed relationship with a vacation or cruise. There are companies that specialize in tours for people with hearing losses. Contact SHHH for more information:
Self Help For Hard Of Hearing People, Inc,
      7910 Woodmont Ave. Suite 1200,
      Bethesda MD 20814-3015,
      301 657 2248, 657 2249 TTY,
      Fax: 301 913 9413;
      E-Mail: national@shhh
      Web: www.shhh.org.
Another source:
      Society for the Advancement of
      Travel for the Handicapped,
      5014 42nd Street NW,
      Washington D.C. 20016,
      202 966-3900.
This is a non-profit organization dedicated to the promotion and improvement of travel and tourism opportunities for the handicapped.

{ 5 }
If Your Spouse, Parent, or Friend Has a Hearing Loss

This chapter is written for those who have frequent contact with someone who has a hearing loss—perhaps a spouse, parent, relative, or close friend. Those of you with a hearing loss would be well advised to keep reading, too, because you may gain some insight into how people who are seemingly insensitive to your problem simply may not know any better. Or maybe they do understand and are having a tough time because you are not facing up to your own hearing loss.

Those of you who do not have a hearing loss: Do you know what it would be like? Chances are, you probably don't. Here's why: You can imagine what it's like to be blind by closing your eyes or turning off the lights, but you can't stop your hearing. Even plugging your ears tightly simulates only a mild hearing loss, and there are distortion factors that normal-hearing people cannot duplicate.

Persons with normal hearing also may ask why such a big deal is made of emotional problems in relation to hearing loss (and why three of the first four chapters of this book dealt with it exclusively).

The most effective way to explain is by illustration.

Here are some of the problems faced by hearing impaired people:

• *Frustration*, because they don't understand much

of what is being said, and have to ask people to repeat themselves.

• *Low self-esteem/confidence*, because they are no longer a perfect whole person and cannot do what others can or what they used to do.

• *Fear of embarrassment*, because they make some inappropriate responses during conversation, or make no response at all when one is expected.

• *Tension*, because they must constantly be extremely alert, afraid they will miss something important, or that someone will change the topic and they won't catch on quickly.

• *Exhaustion*, because for them listening is not a passive activity. It requires that they actively attempt to fill in what they miss, and predict what will be said.

Here are some comparable situations that would make a normal-hearing person experience these feelings:

• *Frustration.* You are buying vegetables at a market in an ethnic neighborhood. You are asking questions of the grocer, who has a very thick accent. Most people around you are speaking a foreign language. You are having a great deal of trouble understanding the grocer, and people behind you in line are growing impatient. The grocer (an arrogant sort of fellow) seems amused that you must continually ask him to repeat himself. He gestures to friends nearby, and says something you do not understand. Everybody—except you—laughs at what the grocer says.

• *Fear of embarrassment.* It's difficult to come up with a directly comparable situation, but you may have experienced this emotion at a party with people you do not know. They may have been part of a different social class, or members of a political or fraternal group you are not part of. When people ask you direct questions, you are afraid of inadvertently offending someone, or displaying ignorance of the topic at hand.

• *Low self-esteem*: You are with a group of people who work and play with computers, but you know nothing about them. As the conversation turns to computer topics, you fall silent and escape as soon as possible.

• *Tension*: You are driving to an appointment in an unfamiliar city; you are alone in the car and it is snowing. You are driving slowly—much to the displeasure of drivers behind you—because you are afraid you'll miss a street sign. You're expending no more physical energy than you would driving home from work in your home town, but how do your nerves feel in this situation?

• *Exhaustion*: You've taken someone to a restaurant for a business meeting. As you begin dinner, a rock band (which you didn't know was going to be there when you picked out the restaurant) starts to play at full blast, of course. You must strain to catch every word, and you find yourself staring at your companion's mouth, trying to get some clue as to what is being said. By the end of the evening, you are tired and irritable. Your pleasant dinner meeting was turned into a real chore because communication was so difficult.

Get the picture? What to you is simple communication is a tiring effort for those with a hearing problem, and the kinds of factors illustrated make it a tedious and trying process. That's why some hearing impaired people tend to forego communication altogether, or can only tolerate some social situations for a brief period of time.

You can take this a step further and try a few hands-on homework assignments to allow you to experience a bit of the world of someone with a hearing loss:

1. Go to a store and tell a clerk that you have a hearing loss and need to have everything written down.
2. Wear earplugs and earmuffs at the same time and try staying alone at night or walking down a street alone.
3. Wear an unusual outfit that you think draws attention and walk around in public. (People wearing hearing aids often feel this way even though others don't usually notice the aids.)
4. Go up to the speaker at a meeting and ask that they speak louder and clearer for you.
5. Turn the television volume to a level where you can just barely hear and then listen to it for a long period of time.
6. Talk to someone on the telephone with the television turned up loudly right next to you.

It is doubly frustrating for the hearing impaired person when their families and friends don't understand how difficult these types of situations can be. In fact, people with hearing losses often feel (with justification) that they are victims of widespread prejudice and misconception. (It's not unheard of for someone with a hearing loss to use the term "bigot" to describe a person who makes no effort to understand the problem.)

Are you treating someone unfairly? Take this brief quiz and find out. Do you:

• Ever talk as if the hearing impaired person isn't there?
• Avoid sitting down to carry on a conversation?
• Leave them out of conversations or activities?
• Just drop a subject with a "never mind" rather then take the time to repeat?
• Make fun of mistakes due to poor hearing?

• Withdraw affection when you are angry over their not hearing?
• Accuse someone with a hearing loss of only listening when he or she wants to?
• Shout if someone doesn't hear the first time?
• Tell someone to turn up their hearing aids?
• Speak to the person as if he or she were a child?
• Take over responsibility for answering the door or the telephone, without being asked to?

If you answered affirmatively to any of these questions, you might be acting very unfairly. Some of the situations need no explanation, and deal with consideration and manners (talking around or ignoring someone in a conversation), while others involve misconceptions that may lead to inappropriate reactions on your part.

For instance, nothing makes a hearing impaired person's blood boil faster than the familiar accusation that "you only listen when you want to—you use your hearing as an excuse to tune out when you're not interested." This holds just a kernel of truth: As has been pointed out, listening is an active (as opposed to a passive) activity for people with a hearing loss. They must make a special effort to understand. What they understand often hinges on a complex mixture of listening conditions, background noise, and the voice of the person speaking; if you take the time to sit down and analyze each particular situation, there will be definite reasons why someone can hear in some situations, but not in others. Yes, it sometimes depends on interest—but if you had to make a tiring effort every time you had to listen, wouldn't you "tune out" from time to time?

Equally rankling is the command to "turn up your hearing aids if you can't understand!" First of all, most people with a sensorineural hearing loss have problems with both sensitivity and discrimination (see Chapter 1) and often hear speech as distorted sound. *Turning up the volume cannot make distorted sound any clearer, and may actually make the situation worse.* Overly loud sound coming through the hearing aids can be unpleasant or even painful, and will certainly be distorted even more. Because of this property of ears and hearing aids, shouting doesn't help someone understand; you may hurt their ears, but that's about all.

Remember, too, that even when someone wears hearing aids and becomes skilled in lipreading, they still will not be able to function precisely in the same manner as someone with good hearing. These issues are addressed elsewhere in this book, but to summarize for you significant others, here are a few facts:

> • Using just one hearing aid causes a "bad side" and gives problems in telling the location of a speaker, which impedes lipreading. It also makes hearing in background noise more difficult.
> • Hearing aids are used on impaired ears—they cannot make the ears normal again. Thus, the result with the aid is limited by the severity of the hearing loss.
> • Hearing losses affect much more than just the loudness of sounds. There is distortion of various kinds. Hearing aids can make sound louder, but they cannot eliminate most of the distortion.
> • Most hearing aids help the least in the situations where they are needed the most—in background noise. If you turn up the aid, you turn up the noise. See chapter 6 for more on this.
> • If sound must travel across distance to the microphone of the hearing aids, it loses power, becomes distorted, and picks up background noise. So get close to the listener.
> • Hearing aids are only as good as the professional who fits them. Also, visits to that professional must

be made for fitting modifications and for periodic "tune ups."
• Lipreading is not an exact science and is very limited.
• Only 30% of English sounds are easily visible on the lips and many of those look alike.
• The shape of sounds on the lips changes with context and with the speaker.
• Lips are not visible in many situations.

There are some materials available to help you understand living with hearing loss. One of the best is first hand experience articles in the SHHH journal (which is sent with membership) about what it is like to live with hearing loss. These can be a real eye opener for those who think hearing loss is a small part of one's life.

Some good books, audio tapes and videotapes are:

Books:

Missing Words: The Family Handbook On Adult Hearing Loss by K. Thomsett & E. Nickerson

What's That Pig Outdoors? by H. Kiser.

Audio tapes

"Say What? An Introduction To Hearing Loss," from The American Academy Of Audiology (@$13), which explains hearing loss and simulates some sentences and words as heard with a hearing loss.

"Sound Hearing, Or Hearing What You Miss," from SHHH @$9 which simulates listening with hearing loss to music, stories, and other situations.

"The Hearing Counseling Kit," Eleanor Stromberg (1997) from Interactive Therapeutics Inc. P.O. Box 1805 Stow, OH 44224-0805. This kit includes a tape that simulates hearing loss in many common situations under different noise and distance conditions.

At $80, it is a bit pricey, but you might borrow it from an audiology facility.

Video tape

"Getting The Most Out Of Your Hearing Aids," by C.E. Koop from SHHH (@$20) gives a realistic view of wearing hearing aids.

You're now aware of what you should not do when dealing with someone with impaired hearing; there are some helpful suggestions about what you should do to enhance communication with your hard-of-hearing spouse, parent, or friend. This list is not all-inclusive, but it reflects feelings of many hearing impaired people about what others could do to make life easier for them.

• Before talking, get their attention first through touching, calling their name, etc.

• Speak in a normal tone of voice, or one that is slightly louder than usual. Don't shout. Make an effort to speak clearly and articulate well, but don't exaggerate your mouth and lip movements. Exaggerating lip movements actually distorts the sounds and makes it more difficult. Because people are not used to seeing such movements, they have no practice reading them. Be precise, but don't overdo it.

• Try to hold your head still while talking, and don't make extraneous gestures, which can distract attention from the message.

• Don't speak rapidly, but don't slow your speech down to the point where it may seem insulting or downright silly.

• Pause frequently between phrases and sentences to allow the listener to catch up.

• Keep your pitch reasonably low. A lower-pitched voice is easier to understand. Also, try to project from the diaphragm and be sure to open your mouth a reasonable amount when you talk (in other words, don't mumble with your teeth closed).

• Don't smile too much. Smiles are wonderful to make the world brighter, but they can distort the mouth while speaking.

• Don't cover your mouth. Keep hands, pens, papers, food, cigarettes, and gum away while speaking. If you have a moustache/beard, keep it trimmed, and take off those dark glasses.

• Try and position yourself where the light falls on your face when speaking; never stand with your back to a window or lamp.

• Face each other when you talk—don't be doing other things at the same time—don't talk when you are busy.

• Don't talk around corners, i.e., from other rooms.

• Alert people to topic changes. It is very tough to lipread and fill in words when you don't know the subject of conversation.

• Give important words separately—like names and places.

• Use appropriate facial expressions, gestures, and other body language.

• Summarize important points.

• Look for signs of uncertainty in the listener.

• Be aware that someone with a hearing impairment will be excessively bothered by background noise (even a little bit of it). So try not to have a television (use the mute button), radio, or other appliance going in the background. Understand that hearing may be difficult in a room full of people.

If you are still not understood correctly, try these repair strategies:

Repeat once—using the same words.
• "Do you want anything at the store?"
• "Let's go to the Irish pub for dinner."
• "I go to an exercise class every morning at the YMCA."

Rephrase—using different words.

- "Can I get you something at the market?"
- "Would you like dinner at the Irish pub tonight?"
- "Each morning I go to the YMCA for aerobics class."

Use two sentences.

- "I'm going to the store. Do you need anything?"
- "Do you want to go out to dinner? How about the Irish pub?"
- "I go to the YMCA every day. I attend an exercise class."

Give the key words separately.

- "Want...anything...store"
- "Dinner...Irish pub...tonight"
- "Exercise...YMCA...morning"

Spell or write the key words.

- I as in ice, R as in rat, S as in so, H as in hair, etc.
- Y as in yellow, M as in Mary, C as in cat, A as in awful.

Some other things that would probably be appreciated:

- Let your hearing impaired significant other know that you want to learn as much as possible about their experience so you can share it with them and help find solutions.
- Talk to the audiologist about what your significant other can and cannot hear.
- Go to the hearing aid appointments with them. Practice lipreading with them and even offer to go to therapy. Encourage them to be assertive. Try out assistive devices with them.
- Troubleshoot difficult communication situations and make suggestions for improving listening environments.
- Be honest in a sensitive way about how their loss affects your life.
- Because listening is a chore for those with hearing

loss, they must take time to rest, especially in a strenuous communication situation such as a party (with multiple speakers and a lot of background noise). If someone wants to be alone for a while, or retreat to a quiet room, accept that decision—don't make an issue of it. People who do this aren't anti-social. They are just tired, and need a break.

There is another important point we should emphasize: Although any family member or friend (significant others) can feel the impact of having a loved one with hearing loss, usually the spouse most acutely feels it. It is the spouse who frequently is over burdened by repeating things endless times, listening to a blasting television, being asked to make telephone calls, acting as interpreter for things not understood, passing up activities that might have been fun or entertaining, limiting friends, and by giving up deep significant discussions, daily small talk, sweet nothings—in fact all but essential messages.

One of the most common questions asked of audiologists by significant others goes something like this:

Why won't my husband/wife/mother/father/friend even think about getting hearing aids? We don't go out anymore and our friends and family complain about him/her. (S)he plays the television so loudly I can't stand it. (S)he has millions of excuses why (s)he didn't hear something and keeps saying there is nothing wrong with his/her hearing. Some days I just want to scream! This is the worst challenge to our relationship yet.

The underlying reasons for not admitting to hearing loss were discussed in Chapter 2. And if no loss is admitted, hearing aids don't seem necessary. What is discussed here is what significant others can do to either get them to see the need for aids, or better cope with a situation that doesn't change.

There is an excellent book by Dr. Michael Harvey, a psychologist, called *Odyssey Of Hearing Loss* (1998), which includes a chapter called, "Presbycusis, Mortality and Brussels Sprouts." It wonderfully describes the trials of adult children trying to talk their mother into wearing her hearing aids. The mother's side of all this is illuminating: to her, the hearing aids are just one step closer to dependence on her children and then to the grave. Trying to force their use only emphasizes the children's growing dominance.

Getting hearing aids involves more than a logical decision such as shopping for a car or a coat. It involves a value and attitude change—both of which take time and lots of emotional as well as intellectual energy. The person obtaining the aids must realize that the devices are not a sign of aging and dependence. They will not result in devaluation of them by others, causing loss of self-esteem. In fact, aids can reduce communication difficulties and thus will not restrict, but will expand their lifestyle and allow them to stay involved. To make hearing aids a positive experience, the benefits of increased socialization and decreased isolation must be seen to outweigh the monetary cost and the energy required for a value/attitude change.

There are many reasons why people reject hearing aids. Frankly, hardly anyone *wants* to wear hearing aids or to spend a lot of money and time unless they are sure it will help. Price is the most common reason given by the person with the loss. However, more likely reasons include:

- Failure to admit to their own loss because day to day changes in hearing are usually minimal
- Stigma of being inferior, unintelligent, less attractive, or less competent with an aid
- Not remembering how important hearing is in their life

• Being told by a physician that they don't need an aid or that "nerve deafness" can't be helped
• Thinking the hearing aids, along with canes, walkers, chair lifts, etc., are just one step closer to the grave
• Rebelling against people (often their children) running their lives and telling them what to do
• Being told by dissatisfied hearing aid users that aids "just don't work," advice often based on people fitted years ago and not with new technology

The average time between a person first noticing a loss and finally going for help is about ten years! Sometimes the best motivation is guiding the person towards the conclusion that wearing aids are in their best interests and those of their family. There are many factors that can affect motivation to get hearing aids. Some can be impacted by significant others.

• **Self-concept issues**. Reassure them that you care about the person, not the hearing. They are loved regardless of their hearing loss, but because you care, you would like to be able to talk to them easily.
• **Attitude toward other hearing aid users**. If significant others make negative comments about other people with hearing loss or hearing aids, it will be generalized back to your loved one. "Old Mrs. Jones is deaf even with those huge hearing aids." "Does Ralph have to get hearing aids? I didn't think he was that old." "She wears two hearing aids and still can't hear a thing."
• **Availability of communication partners**. If you never go anywhere, you don't need a car. If you don't have anyone to talk to, you don't need hearing aids. As it gets harder and harder to communicate with someone, we tend to avoid them. That person needs to know that there are people who want to talk to

them and hearing aids will make it a lot easier on both of you. The extent to which a person keeps frequent contact with significant others can seriously impact the effect of a hearing loss and the success of hearing aids—not to mention general health.

• **The frequency of communication demands**. The acts that seem kindest to us may be the ones that allow the person to deny the hearing loss forever. If the significant other talks loudly, repeats habitually without comment, turns the television loud enough to drive others out, and isolates themselves and their loved one from the normally hearing world, the need for hearing aids will not be as obvious. Your being a martyr doesn't really help the person with the hearing loss. It encourages the denial of hearing loss.

What can you do, then? First, although it seems a bit cruel, you need to resist the desire to automatically compensate for the loss all of the time. It must be made clear that everyone else is having to make a real effort because communication is becoming a big problem. Only then will there be motivation. That doesn't mean that nagging is a good idea. You can set up the situation so they come to the realization themselves. It serves as a gentle reminder that you care enough to want easy communication with one you love. Once that person has gotten hearing aids and counseling, keep those compensatory skills handy because there still won't be normal hearing and the help is occasionally appropriate.

Try generating with your significant other a list of pros and cons of wearing hearing aids. The pros will usually win out. Or try asking, "What would happen if you decided to try hearing aids? What bad things? What good things?"

Probably the best thing you can learn is clear

speech. It is easy with a little practice and it can increase understanding by 15-20%. Clear speech means:

- Accurate, precise, fully formed sounds
- A little louder, but still natural
- Slowing speech by adding frequent pauses at natural places
- Emphasis of key words that carry the main meaning
- Lively inflection and stress

It sounds tough at first, but with a little practice, it soon comes naturally.

Continue your social activities as much as possible, even if your significant other refuses to participate with you. This could be incentive for them to get help so they can join you. Get a set of good earplugs to wear when the television or stereo are on loud. It will make it more tolerable for you, and might be a big hint for someone else. Get to know someone who is successfully wearing hearing aids (ask an audiologist to introduce you). Once you get to know them, introduce them to your spouse/parent/friend. This person may be able to talk with personal knowledge about the doubts, fears, and reservations of getting hearing aids.

As a significant other without hearing loss, it is difficult to know how you "should react" when faced with having a loved one with a loss. Do you ignore it and not talk about it so they don't get hurt or upset? Should you pity them, cry with them, or try to see the humor in the situation? If you are very hesitant, be aware that your reactions are probably not those of an inconsiderate, intolerant, selfish person. They are probably those of millions of others in your situation. Let's look at typical significant other emotional responses.

Concern:
"I get very upset when other people make comments under their breath about my brother."

"I'd like to talk to her about her hearing problem but don't want to make a big thing and embarrass her."

Anxiety:

"I worry that he won't hear a car coming or someone breaking into the house."

"If we're the same age, and she has all these problems hearing, when will it be my turn?"

Embarrassment:

"When we go out, people will think he's crazy or stupid."

"When she makes a silly comment, everyone looks at me as if they feel sorry for me because I have to live with her."

Frustration:

"I just want life to be like it was when we got married. It was so easy before he got this hearing problem."

"I want so badly to help Dad, but he won't get hearing aids."

Annoyance:

"It drives me crazy when she takes her hearing aids off at night and she can't hear me at all."

"Everything just takes so much more time because of the hearing loss."

Impatience:

"Forget what I said, it's not worth it."

"I already told you that a thousand times!"

Sadness:

"I guess Mom will never be able to enjoy her grandkids because she can't hear them."

"I can see how hurt my mom is when my dad ridicules her about her hearing loss."

Anger:
> "When she doesn't hear me, something just snaps inside me and I start to shout at her even though I know it makes it worse."

> "Why can't my father be like other dads?"

Guilt and incompetence:
> "I should help, but I can't fix it."

> "I want so badly to stop his hurting, but I am worthless."

Probably the best response is open communication and sharing about the hearing loss. Those with hearing loss may rationalize, "If others can talk about it without embarrassment, it can't be that bad. But if they can't even speak about it, having a hearing loss must be a terrible thing."

Here are some questions commonly asked by family and friends of hearing impaired people.

You say it's important for the light to be on my face so someone can see my mouth. Well, my father has never had lipreading lessons, so why should I bother?
Lipreading (which will be discussed in Chapter 11) is something everyone does, without any special training—although training can make these skills much more efficient. You lipread too, when you're trying to follow a conversation in heavy background noise. See for yourself, the next time you're in such a situation. Try to understand speech without looking at faces.

When I talk with my hearing impaired husband, I can repeat myself several times, but he still doesn't understand. What do I do then?
If a person does not understand after one repeti-

tion, there must be some sounds in the phrase that can't be heard with their hearing loss. It is unlikely that more repetitions will change that. There are several strategies, mentioned above, that you can employ when a hearing impaired person does not understand you. For example, when you do repeat, make sure you are looking directly at the person and use clear (but not distorted) diction. Also, it often helps to use a synonym for an important word in your sentence, for it may often be only one word that the person to whom you're speaking doesn't understand. For example, if you can't connect with the sentence, "It's really hot in the kitchen," try, "It's really warm in the kitchen." If you still have no luck, try another related term: "It's really warm working near the stove." Finally, consider breaking up the statement into two sentences. This is much easier for a hearing impaired person to figure out. If you weren't understood when you said, "Are you going to sing in church today?" try, "I am going to church today. Are you going to sing?"

If people can learn to read lips, why do they still have trouble understanding?

The amount of information that can be picked up by reading lips has been greatly overestimated, especially by mystery writers who portray a character that reads lips through binoculars, for example. Perhaps someone with truly exceptional abilities can pick up the thread of a conversation through visual cues alone, but for almost everyone else it is extremely difficult. There are many speech sounds that simply cannot be detected visually. See the limitations of lipreading listed previously.

Is it possible that my husband uses his hearing loss to not pay attention to what I say?

Despite all the jokes about husbands having selective hearing, it is critical to any relationship to be aware of the difference between not paying attention and being unable to hear. A person with a hearing loss will find it harder to "tune in" to those around him because listening is an active process that requires a certain level of attention and mental energy. It is impossible to maintain a high level of both continuously. If the process of trying to understand the speech is very difficult, there may not be much mental energy left to commit the information to memory. So, when questioned later, it may seem like not paying attention. Try getting his attention by calling his name and making sure he is looking at you. Then, when finished, ask if he has understood you.

The next chapter will (like the rest of the book) be directed toward those with a hearing loss, but normal-hearing readers who were persuaded to read this chapter might want to continue. Hearing aids, covered in Chapter 6, may be subject to more myth and misunderstanding than any other aspect of hearing impairment.

{ 6 }
The Hearing Aid

This chapter may seem somewhat out of order, coming after a long section on emotional problems and before a discussion of doctors, audiologists, and hearing aid dispensers. However, it is in the middle of the book for a reason. There is a strong temptation to think of a hearing aid as the first step in solving problems associated with a hearing loss. It is not. As we've seen in previous chapters, emotional acceptance of the problem, and a willingness to do something about it, come first.

Only 20-25 percent of the 28 million Americans with hearing losses own hearing aids! Yet, a hearing aid is the single most important thing you can do for your hearing loss. Only a very small percentage cannot benefit at least some from aids if they are willing to learn.

It is also common to think of hearing aids as the end process in coping with a hearing loss. That's certainly not true, either. Diligent practice with aids, hearing therapy, counseling, and a good attitude must go hand-in-hand with wearing aids.

That's why the discussion of hearing aids is in the middle of the book. Getting hearing aids is, actually, somewhere in the middle of the process of coping with a hearing loss.

Many of you are wearing hearing aids now, but are not happy with them. Some of you have never worn aids, and would like some specific information on the various models and the benefits they offer. Still others may have worn a hearing aid for a while and given up on it. If that's the case, your problems may have stemmed from lack of knowledge about what an aid can and cannot do. Let's first consider those benefits and limitations.

Hearing aids can...

...make soft sound louder, bringing speech to a more comfortable level for listening. Simply because of the increase in loudness, your under-standing of speech will be improved.

...allow you to hear in some situations that used to give you trouble, such as in church. Even though aids might not enable you to hear every word of a distant speaker, you will pick up more sounds. These sounds will serve as cues to enable you to fill in the parts you miss, possibly through lipreading.

...help you to hear high–pitched sounds, such as bird calls. Not only do high–pitched sounds give you more of a "live" feeling (being in touch with the world around you), they also aid in your ability to understand speech.

...help you to feel more at ease in social situations, by making it easier for you to understand what's being said. The aid can also alert people to the fact that you don't hear well, and this may induce them to make an extra effort when communicating with you. If you still attach a stigma to hearing loss, this may be hard for you to accept; if so a simple change in hairstyle will camouflage most aids. The newer completely-in-the-canal aids are almost invisible.

Hearing aids cannot:

...enable you to hear extremely soft sounds. If the

hearing aids were set so you could hear all the very soft sounds that a normal-hearing person could detect, louder sounds would blast intolerably. Some of the newer circuits can help, but even with hearing aids that work perfectly, you will still have the equivalent of a slight loss.

…cure distortion. The aids only modify sound going into your ear. If your inner ear and brain distort sound (causing difficulty in discrimination, the ability to understand), the hearing aids will help somewhat just by making the sound louder. But even though the sound is louder, the aids can't eliminate the distortion; they can only make the distorted sound louder and give you a better chance of figuring it out.

…restore a completely natural sound. Hearing aids are, after all, digital, electrical and mechanical devices, and therefore will slightly change the quality of what you hear, just as a radio does. Because it's a relatively small instrument, the aid cannot amplify all frequencies; music, for example, will not retain all of its rich harmonics. In fact, what sounds natural to you, may not be what normal hearing people hear. You've had a hearing loss for awhile, and your "natural" is not true sound anymore. The sound from the hearing aid may be better for you to hear speech than the sound you consider to be natural.

…allow you to hear well when there is a lot of background noise or many people talking all at once. By adjusting the volume of your aids you may hear better, but these are the situations where the aids will be of least help to you. The aids cannot amplify only what you want to hear and ignore the noise. You will need to rely on your lipreading again. There is new technology for listening in background noise, though, and we'll cover that later in this chapter.

...amplify only what you want to hear. The aid will also amplify background noise, the sound of your own footsteps, appliance motors running, the sounds of yourself chewing, and a few other body noises that you didn't know others could hear. You probably haven't heard these sounds normally in quite some time because of the gradual onset of your hearing loss, and it will take some time to adjust to hearing them well again.

So what are realistic expectations of hearing aids?
• Performance in quiet and in noise should be better than unaided, but, in noise will not be as good as in quiet.

•Soft speech should be heard, average speech should be comfortable, and loud speech not uncomfortable nor distorted.

• The sound of your own voice should be acceptable.

• There should be no feedback (whistling or squealing) at comfortable loudness levels.

• The aids should expand the range of environments in which you can hear, but not to all environments.

• There should be no physical pain or discomfort.

To sum up: Hearing aids cannot restore normal hearing. They can, however, help you make the most of what hearing you have. You can usually function in a fairly normal way even though you don't hear normally.

Having said this, we should note that satisfaction with hearing aids has increased tremendously with the new technology available. There is still an 8% return rate on all types of hearing aids. The primary reasons are: unrealistic expectations, fitting of old technology aids, less qualified dispensers, and not enough orientation and follow up. Hopefully this book will help you learn what to expect and allow you to better evaluate dispensers. Be sure to demand follow up, as you are paying for it. Optional counseling takes at least 1-2 hours and several sessions of orientation are even better. Of course those people with a positive attitude, high motivation, willingness to try, ability to adapt, and a feeling of control over their lives are most successful. It also helps to have a support network of friends and family who encourage hearing aid use. Realistic expectations play a big part too. Expecting hearing aids to bring 20-year-old hearing to 65-year-old ears is bound to lead to disappointment. Also doomed is the concept of instant optimal benefit from the aids when the brain needs time to adjust to the change. This acclimatization of the brain to the new sound could take weeks, so be patient.

For additional encouragement, recommended reading is: *Consumers Digest,* July/August 1999, an article on high technology hearing aids.

How do hearing aids work?

An aid is divided into several major parts (shown in Figures 6.1 and 6.2), all of which play a role in amplifying

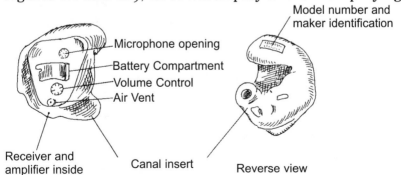

Figure 6.1. Basic parts of an in-the-ear aid.

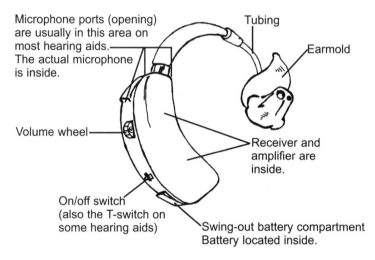

Microphone ports (opening) are usually in this area on most hearing aids. The actual microphone is inside.

Tubing

Earmold

Volume wheel

Receiver and amplifier are inside.

On/off switch (also the T-switch on some hearing aids)

Swing-out battery compartment Battery located inside.

Figure 6.2. Basic parts of a behind-the-ear hearing aid.

sound and directing it into your ear. It is important for you to know something about the structure of the aid, because you are likely to have difficulties from time to time, and a working knowledge of the device can help you solve simple problems and save yourself a great deal of frustration.

The *microphone* picks up sound and turns it into electrical energy. The *battery compartment* holds the battery which powers the aid. The *amplifier*, using the power from the battery, boosts the intensity of the tiny electrical signal from the microphone. The receiver turns the amplified electrical signal back into sound again.

The *canal insert* in the one-piece aid fits into your ear and directs the sound into the ear canal. In the kind of aid that rests behind the ear, an earmold directs the sound into the ear. The *earmold* is a hollow piece of plastic molded specifically for your ear. It extends a half inch or so into the ear canal. It also helps to hold the aid in place. A less obvious function is to seal off the amplified sound in the ear canal so that it does not go back out the canal, back into the microphone and cause a squealing sound, called feedback.

In addition to these basic parts, most hearing aids also come equipped with a volume control to adjust the amount of loudness, just like the volume control on a radio. Most aids also have an on-off switch which may be part of the volume control, although some just disengage the battery to turn it off.

Although all hearing aids have these same basic components, their appearance may vary quite a bit. Different styles have evolved to suit the preferences of various users. This wide assortment often leaves a newcomer feeling somewhat bewildered. However, once you realize that hearing aids fall into one of *five basic styles*— and learn the advantages and limitations of each— things won't seem nearly as confusing.

The basic styles are *in-the-ear, in-the-canal, completely-in-the-canal, behind-the-ear, eyeglass,* and *body aids.* Hearing aids worn on the torso (body aids), or in eyeglass frames are no longer in common use in the United States, but are still used in developing countries. Body aids provide tremendous power with less feedback (squealing), are easy to handle, and are very sturdy. Thus they may be used for infants with profound losses, or geriatrics with vision or manipulation problems. The eyeglass aids have the inconvenience of connecting your vision to your hearing and are difficult to fit, but are used in special fittings where there is only one impaired ear or where feedback is a major problem. Due to their low usage rate, these two styles will not be discussed at length here. Examples of the other types are pictured and described below.

Before discussing the various types of hearing aids, we should point out that the choice of style of aid is not entirely up to you and your cosmetic preferences. The shape of your ear and ear canal may eliminate some styles. Your ability to manipulate small controls may be a factor. There may be medical contra-indications, such as chronic infections in the ear canal, or even an overactive wax producing system that dictates the style. Other factors, of course, are the results of your hearing test such as the degree of hearing loss, and indications of need for special features that take up space.

In-The-Ear Hearing Aids

About 35 percent of hearing aids now sold are in–the–ear types. To manufacture this aid, an impression is made of the ear canal and the bowl–like opening of the outer ear; the components are then built into a plastic case that is molded from the impression.

Figure 6.3. An in–the–ear aid. This fits within the bowl–shaped opening of the outer ear. (Photo courtesy of Widex.)

Advantages. The in-the-ear aid will not interfere with eyeglasses, and many people feel this type of aid is easier to put on and take off than a behind–the–ear style; it may therefore be helpful to people with arthritis or some other problem with manual dexterity.

Limitations. Because they are molded individually, you can't try on in–the–ear aids before you order them. However, with some of the newer technology, the hearing aid dispenser can let you listen to a simulation of the aid in the office.

Because the aid fills up your ear, it may be uncomfortable in hot weather due to sweating. In–the–ear aids are generally reliable, but some people feel they require more repairs than behind–the–ear styles. Repair time poses another problem: If your in–the–ear aid goes in for repair, your loaner will probably be a behind–the–ear model, and you'll need a separate earmold to use it.

Fig. 6.4. An in-the-ear aid in use. (Photo Courtesy of Widex)

In–the–ear (ITE) aids come in two basic sizes, *full concha* and *half-concha* (see Figure 6.4). *Concha* means "bowl," and the term simply means that the full–concha ITE fills the whole bowl–shaped part of the ear, and the half concha ITE fills roughly half the bowl. In fact, the half concha is a good compromise because it has less bulk than the full in-the-ear, yet is still easier to handle than the smaller aids to be described next. The size you get depends partly on your pocketbook (in general, smaller aids cost more because it is more expensive to miniaturize them), the shape of your ear, and your dexterity (smaller aids are harder to insert and harder for you to adjust).

In-The-Canal Aids

In-the–canal (ITC) aids have captured about 25 percent of the market, and their popularity continues to rise. The ITC fits down into the ear canal, with only a small portion extending into the bowl–like area of the ear. The amount of the ITC that fits into the canal depends on how much circuitry goes into the particular aid, and the size of your ear canal. The smaller the ear canal, the more the aid will protrude into the bowl–shaped part of the ear. Figure 6.5 shows an ITC actually in an ear.

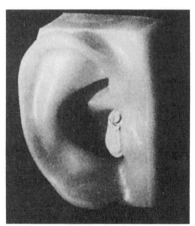

Fig. 6.5. This is an in-the-canal aid.
(Photo Courtesy of Telex
Communications, Inc.)

Advantages. Visibility is the prime advantage; simply stated, a small aid can't be seen as easily. A secondary advantage is the position of the microphone. Since the aid picks up sound farther into the ear canal, it more closely mimics the natural way the ear hears sound, taking advantage of the natural resonance of the ear. Also, wind noise is less of a problem because the microphone is protected by the outer ear.

Limitations. ITC aids can be difficult to handle and insert. The battery is very small, and requires good dexterity and close–up vision to insert. The volume control must be adjusted by touch (you can't see it in a mirror) and you have to stick your finger down in your ear to make the adjustment.

Another limitation is cost. A smaller aid costs more; you are paying for high–tech, super–miniaturized components.

There is also a not-so-obvious reason why the ITC aid is more expensive: Because people often have difficulty handling the tiny instrument, there are more of these aids returned to the manufacturer than other styles. This costs the companies money. Since they—like any other firm—need to make a profit, the cost of the ITC is increased. Usually, the added costs to the manufacturer and dispenser will add up to about an additional $150 over a standard in-the-ear aid.

Another point to consider: ITC aids do not have as much power as other aids. There are several reasons. First, because the microphone is right down in the canal, and the aid is so small, there is a greater likelihood of sound leaking around the aid and feeding back into the microphone; therefore, the amount of amplification simply cannot be as great as other models where the microphone is farther from the part of the aid that emits the amplified sound. You will also have to make more frequent battery changes, since the ITC uses a very tiny battery.

ITC aids also have certain limitations regarding the special features that can be built-in. Larger aids can accommodate a telephone coil (a device to automatically pick up the electrical signals of the telephone) but this is very difficult to engineer into an ITC.

Finally, remember that if you have a very small ear canal, the ITC will stick out into the concha, so why pay extra for an aid that will be visible anyway?

Completely-In-The-Canal-Aids (CIC)

The public asked for an aid that didn't show and the hearing aid industry listened. Fig. 6.6 demonstrates that the aid fits way down inside the ear canal near the eardrum with only a thin plastic handle for removal sticking into the concha.

Unless you use a remote control, there usually is no volume control because you can't reach the aid once it is in place.

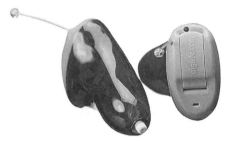

Fig. 6.6. A Completely in-the-Canal Aid. (Photo courtesy of Oticon)

Advantages. There are some other advantages to this style besides cosmetic, such as easier use of telephones, less power needed (the closer to the eardrum the less power needed) so there is decreased feedback and distortion, acoustics that make it easier to tell the direction of a sound, less occlusion effect (the effect you get when you plug your ears and talk), less wind noise, and more amplification of the high pitches.

Limitations. However, this device doesn't come without a few limitations. The inner portion of your ear canal has thin skin so the fitting may be uncomfortable and may have to be done more than once. The fit of this style is critical so you may have to go back a few times. The aids are not powerful enough for severe or profound losses. Some fine manual dexterity is required to use the small device. In fact, it is recommended that you ask to see a model and try putting the battery in and out a few times before you order one.

There may not be room for vents which help in relieving the feelings of pressure that sometimes occur with in-the-canal models. Some ear canals are not big enough or the right shape to hold this style. Experience has shown a higher breakdown rate than with other styles. Also the price is considerably more because of the added expertise required for fitting them. Regardless, this style has already cornered about 20% of the sales and the design is improving all the time.

Behind–the–Ear Hearing Aids

Behind-the-ear hearing aids, such as the one shown in Figure 6.7, were losing popularity and were down to 16% of the sales, but have recently had increased interest. The rise to about 20% is due to the technology that can be included in that size hearing aid, the additional advantage of their dual/directional microphones, and the decreasing stigma about wearing aids.

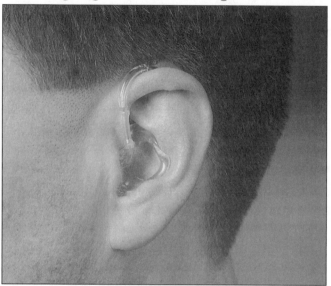

Figure 6.7. A behind-the-ear aid as it is worn.
(Photo courtesy of Oticon Corp.)

This type of aid is encased in a plastic compartment about one to one-and-a-half inches long, and a half inch thick. The aid rests behind the ear, with a hook and a piece of flexible tubing going over the top of the ear and connecting the aid to the earmold. The earmold, depending on its type, extends from one quarter to three quarters of an inch into the ear canal.

Advantages. Behind-the-ear styles are easily interchangeable if one has to go in for service, and are typically used for difficult-to-fit hearing losses, special technology, severe losses, or when someone cannot handle a smaller ITE or ITC aid. These aids usually require less repair since the earmolds take the wear and tear. It's a larger aid, which allows space for more technology and enjoys the most advantage for dual/directional microphones that help hearing in background noise. With most hairstyles the aid itself is not visible and the earmold that may be visible, is very unobtrusive.

Limitations. In a few cases, people with glasses have difficulty wearing a behind-the-ear aid. If the temple of the eyeglasses is exceptionally large, or if the lens prescription is so precise that a slight alteration of position is distracting, a behind-the-ear style may not be advisable. Also, some people just don't have enough space between their ear and the side of their head to accommodate the device.

With all these types of aids to choose from, you should have little trouble finding one that suits your individual needs and preferences. The technology, by the way, is truly marvelous. The hearing aid industry has advanced more in the last ten years than during the previous forty, when the modern hearing aid was being developed. Much of this advancement is due to the space program and advances in computer technology. The search for ways to miniaturize reliable equipment in a space capsule has paid off in many ways, including compact and reliable hearing aids, heart pacemakers implanted in the chest, and the familiar pocket calculator.

High Tech Advances

Although we have mentioned some of the recent advances in hearing aids earlier in this book, below is a summary of some of the options that are now available.

Some of these advances may not be appropriate for you and your loss. Talk to your hearing aid dispenser for advice. You will have to pay for the technology, but most of it is well worth the price.

• *Down sizing of hearing aids.* Some of the CIC aids are very small and fit way down inside the ear with only a tiny transparent handle at the opening of the canal. Even the BTE aids are being made smaller. But remember that there is sometimes a sacrifice in cost, ease of handling, power, and available circuitry. Also, some people don't have the appropriate anatomy for the smaller aids.

• *Noise reduction circuits*, often called automatic signal processing (ASP) circuits. These circuits "sense" the noise and automatically adjust themselves to reduce, but not eliminate, the effects of noise that make it intolerable to listen to. If you could eliminate all the noise, you would also be cutting out the speech because they are often at the same pitches.

Most manufacturers make an ASP aid, but you will get what you pay for, i.e., the more sophisticated ones are quite expensive and even they cannot take away all the noise.

• *Directional/dual microphones.* The ASP helps you to tolerate loud background noise. However, research has shown only one advance in hearing aids that actually helps hearing speech in background noise: directional microphones. First, it's best to have hearing aids that amplify the high pitches of speech if you can hear them. Then the directional microphones pick up and amplify the sound directly in front of you (assuming you look at what you want to hear), much more than the sounds from other directions. Certainly you will hear the noise which is directly in front of you, but the reduction of the rest of the noise will help you to hear the speech because there is less competition from less noise.

It's like the sound system a reporter or sports announcer uses to make their voice heard over the roar of the surrounding crowd. The high tech digital aids use more than one microphone (dual) which works even better. These directional microphones are well worth the extra money. It's a good idea to get a switch so you can turn off the directional effect if you want to hear well from all around you.

The directional effect is best with BTE aids, but is significant with ITE aids as well. It is usually not possible on ITC or CIC aids.

• *Compression circuits.* These circuits were originally designed for people who cannot tolerate loud sounds but they provide easier listening in noise for almost everyone. They reduce their own power once the environment gets loud and then increase the power when soft sounds come through. Some are called wide dynamic range compression (WDRC) which means they make soft sounds audible, conversational sounds comfortable, and loud sounds tolerable as they are not amplified at all. This improves sound quality, comfort and ease of listening.

Multiple compression channels found in the high tech aids means that the speech pitch range is divided into segments (called bands) that process information separately to fit your specific loudness needs in that region—specifically gain, output and/or compression. The analog aids usually have 1-3 bands, the digital up to 15! Your ear may hear quite differently in the low pitches than the highs, so the flexibility is important. This feature can even increase the volume for consonants (soft high pitched sounds which carry the meaning of speech) and reduce volume for vowels (louder low pitched sounds which can overpower consonants).

• *Class D amplifiers.* Almost all current aids now use a class D amplifier, but if you think you are getting a "real deal" on a very low cost aid, it may have one of the old class A's which have more distortion, fewer high pitches and poorer battery life.

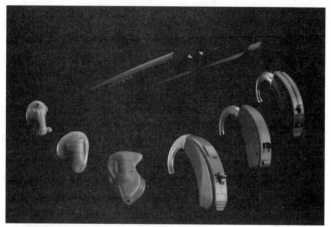

Figure 6.8 Programmable aids with remote contol.
(Photo courtesy GN ReSound)

The digital world.

We can't escape it. The digital computer world has invaded almost every aspect of our lives and is here to stay—for better or for worse. Fortunately, in hearing aids, it seems to be for the better.

In the early 1990's digitally programmable analog hearing aids hit the market. By the end of the 1990's, these programmable aids accounted for about 25% of sales. These analog hearing aids can be fine tuned by a digital computer during the fitting process, to accommodate your hearing loss. Also, most of them have from 2-8 different programs tuned for various situations, which can be accessed with a touch of a button on either the aid itself or on a remote control. So if you aren't hearing well in a situation, you can try a different program that may be more suited to those conditions.

Standard analog hearing aids are usually ineffective in many difficult listening environments, so if you need to hear in lots of situations, these programmable analog aids are a big help. And if you find an environment that none of the programs works for, the aid can be reprogrammed.

If your hearing changes, the aid can be reprogrammed so you don't need to get new aids. These aids come in all styles from BTE to CIC (see fig. 6.8). They are called hybrids because they are analog hearing aids (the same as the old aids) but are digitally programmed by a computer.

These programmable aids have a 13% higher overall satisfaction level. Reported improvements include use in multiple environments, better quality of life, comfort with loud sounds, reduced feedback, and better performance in noise.

The mid 1990's introduced hearing aids that are totally digital, and by the late 90's they made up over 10% of the market. "Digital" is a word that is often used but rarely defined, so let's take a second to nail down the meaning and explore how a digital aid works. These aids convert the speech signal into electrical impulses that can be manipulated by a digital signal processor (DSP) in ways that cannot be done with analog aids, which use automatic signal processing (ASP). A converter then changes the signals back into clearer, cleaner sounds.

In the older analog aids the person was fit to the hearing aid, but with digital technology the hearing aid is fit to the person. Adjustments that become necessary as a hearing loss changes or the person's lifestyle changes, can be done in a brief office visit. The aids can have special features like noise reduction systems, compression systems, dual microphones, low battery warnings, feedback reduction systems, and digital cell phone compatibility. And there is no circuit noise; i.e., the humming sound of an analog hearing aid that annoys those whose hearing is fairly good in the low pitches.

But keep in mind that at this point the technology seems to have outdistanced our ability to utilize it. That is, we aren't using it to its fullest potential. Digital aids will eventually improve the speech understanding abilities of more people in more listening conditions than any analog aid. They are not, however, always necessary for everyone; the choice depends on your lifestyle, your hearing loss and your communication needs. There are certain hearing aid features that are usually recommended by most audiologists such as compression technology, binaural aids, a strong properly oriented telecoil, and dual/directional microphones. But beyond these factors, the choices are individually determined.

Many people are intimidated by the concept of digital technology and associate it with bad past experiences with computers, VCR's , microwaves, and so forth. Actually the all digital hearing aids are some of the easiest to use. You don't even need to worry about a volume control. It's a "set it and forget it" deal. The analog hybrid programmable aids take more manipulation and learning, but once you get the hang of it, they are not difficult to use.

Remote controls. (see fig. 6.8) Some people are embarrassed to adjust the volume of their hearing aids in public, or they cannot manipulate the tiny controls on the aids. Remote controls were developed to help change programs on the hybrid aids mentioned above, but they are also useful for unobtrusive adjustment, and easy manipulation. They are, however, easy to lose or forget. You also need a place to put them—pockets help.

Implantable hearing aids. Not to be confused with

the cochlear implant described below, these are hearing aids which are actually surgically implanted somewhere in the head. They are not appropriate in most cases and are a very drastic step. But since the research and development in this area is growing, we'll include some more specific information.

There are several versions of this type of aid. The least complex is based on the adhesion of titanium and bone tissue and replaces the cumbersome bone conduction aids mentioned below. A titanium screw is surgically implanted in the skull above the outer ear with part of it sticking through the skin. Then a sound processor with a microphone is attached. The screw vibrates the skull, bypassing an abnormal or infection prone outer or middle ear and sends the sound directly to a relatively normal inner ear.

In the other aids, the electronics are surgically implanted somewhere under the skin around the ear with a connection that drives the bones in the middle ear. The connection to the outside microphone may be through an opening in the skin or transmitted across the intact skin.

The latter type of implanted aids can be used with sensorineural (inner ear) hearing losses. The advantages over regular aids are: better sound quality, low visibility, comfort, no feedback, and more gain in the high pitches. But, consider that against: a surgical procedure that may need to be repeated every few years, some restrictions on the type of ear and hearing loss, relatively high cost, and periodic recharging.

Tactile aids. These aids use the sense of touch on the skin of the arm, fingers, chest, or stomach to decipher speech. They are for those whose hearing loss is so severe that they cannot use a conventional hearing aid.

Cochlear implants. A fairly new development in the area of help is the cochlear implant. In this expensive, but fairly safe, surgical procedure, over 20 electrodes are inserted into the inner ear (cochlea). After the surgery has healed, the person wears a small electronic device on the upper body that analyzes the sound picked up by a microphone near the ear. The resulting signal is sent to the electrodes in the inner ear (through an opening in the skin or transmitted across intact skin), which directly stimulates the auditory nerve and bypasses severely damaged hair cells.

The media have done a great job of publicizing this new technique, even calling it a "bionic ear". What they may not tell you is, first of all, that the surgery will destroy parts of the inner ear, so only people who are severely hard of hearing or profoundly deaf, get little if any benefit from hearing aids, and have nothing to lose are selected for surgery. But as the research develops these implants, they are being tried on adults with less and less of a degree of loss. However, it will be a long time before those with mild or moderate losses can get more help from an implant than from hearing aids.

A second very important fact is that the procedure often does not bring back the ability to understand speech without the help of lipreading, although it certainly makes lipreading a lot easier. Many people, however, can carry on a conversation quite well and some can even communicate over the telephone after this procedure. For almost all, the device puts the person back in touch with an auditory world.

A third factor to consider is the extensive pre-surgical testing, post-surgical fitting, and rehabilitation that must be done for success with the device. It may involve many fitting adjustment sessions as well as therapy to train your ears and brain to use the new signal. Adults usually get some improvement right away, but they require weeks of training for optimal success. All of this can cost up to $50,000, but some insurances will pay.

Care of Hearing Aids

There's another effect of these recent technological breakthroughs: Hearing aid users are now buying new aids on the average of one every three years because they want to take advantage of more modern, increasingly sophisticated models. A hearing aid certainly can be expected to last longer than three years, but eventually will wear out and have to be replaced.

Why? Because hearing aids are extremely delicate pieces of equipment, and get pretty rough handling. On top of this, consumers demand that aids be small—which makes them less durable—and that they be relatively inexpensive. Manufacturers probably could build a hearing aid that would last a lifetime, but it would be prohibitively expensive (not that an aid is cheap, now; costs will be discussed more fully in Chapter 9).

With reasonable care, a hearing aid can last five years or so; longer if you're meticulous about proper handling, care, and maintenance. Here are some suggestions on how to preserve what is, after all, a substantial investment:

- Be careful of moisture. Keep the aid away from steamy kitchens or bathrooms where someone has just taken a hot shower. Also, be careful not to hit the aid with hair spray, or other aerosols. Getting caught in the rain won't do your hearing aid any good, but droplets of water aren't as harmful as vapor. Usually, your hair or a hat will keep rain water from harming the aid. Never wear the aid while bathing.
- Don't expose the aid to intense heat. Leaving it on the window-sill in bright sunshine can damage it, as can setting the aid on top of a radiator.
- Protect it from shock. Don't handle the aid roughly, and never set it where it could be knocked to the floor.

• Protect it from dust. Small dust particles can clog up the openings to the microphone. Remove the aid when you are in dusty environments.

• The earmold or the canal opening of the in-the-ear aid may sometimes get wax lodged in the small holes in the part that goes down into the ear. If the wax is near the edge of the hole, carefully pick the wax out with a pin or toothpick, being careful not to damage the opening. In fact it's a good idea to check every morning for any wax and pick it out. In the evening when the wax is soft it may be pushed down and won't come out as one piece. Just be sure you do this procedure with the aid turned up side down so a piece of wax does not fall down inside the aid. The only other cleaning you need to do is using a cloth or tissue to wipe off the outside surface. If you are prone to ear canal infections, wipe off the outside with disposable disinfectant wipes which are available in a canister from the drug store.

• If the wax has worked its way farther into the opening of an earmold of a BTE you can clean this yourself. Disconnect the earmold and the flexible tubing from the BTE hearing aid itself. Just carefully pull it apart—you won't break anything. *Don't pull* the earmold and the tubing apart; they are glued together. Now that the earmold and tubing are disconnected from the aid, soak them in warm water. (Never use hot water because you will melt the glue that bonds them.) Then, rinse the earmold and connecting tube with clean water, dry them thoroughly, and fit them back on the aid. Be sure it is oriented in the correct direction.

If wax becomes lodged farther into the opening of an in-the-ear aid, you must see your hearing aid dispenser for professional cleaning.

If you produce lots of wax, talk to the dispenser about getting a "wax guard," a small screen that can be changed by you or the dispenser. The screen will catch wax before it becomes impacted into the aid. Some manufacturers have other types of wax management systems.

• Once a year, have the aid cleaned and checked by your dealer or dispenser (there's a distinction, which will be explained in Chapter 9, but both terms refer to the person who sold you the aid).

• Wax plugging up the hole in an ITE or ITC aid is one of the more common problems, and repair can cost around a hundred dollars if the unit has to go back to the manufacturer for service.

Adjusting to Hearing Aids

There are common problems you may encounter when adjusting to the hearing aids. Don't forget that you will need an adjustment period; you need to "break in" the aids, just like you'd adjust to a new pair of shoes. A common problem associated with hearing aids is encountered when people put new aids in and attempt to wear them full time through all sorts of conditions, which is something like buying those new shoes and immediately taking a ten–mile hike.

Here are some points to keep in mind:

• If you have worn aids before and are buying new ones, don't expect the new aids to sound exactly like the old ones. Don't keep switching back and forth to compare. Just put the old aids in a drawer and keep them for spares when your new ones need repair.

• Everyone's adjustment period is not the same. It is a mistake to assume that you will adjust as quickly or as slowly as your friend. The average adjustment time is two to four weeks, but this varies widely. Keep in mind that your brain needs time to make full use of this new information.

• The first thing you'll have to adjust to is the sound of your own voice. If you've never worn aids before, the sound of your voice may come as a shock, since you're used to hearing your voice conducted to your hearing mechanism through your bones. Now, you are hearing through microphones in your hearing aids—sort of like hearing yourself on a tape recorder. So when you first get the aids, read out loud to yourself at home in order to get used to the new sound of your voice.

• You also must become used to hearing other people's voices through the microphones of the aids. Any time you listen to a voice through a synthetic instrument the tonal quality will be different. The aids actually are changing the tonal quality, accentuating the high pitches. But in addition to giving greater clarity to sound, those high pitches also can sound "tinny" and be irritating. Essentially, then, you're getting used to a new sound. You will adjust, but it will take time.

• There are many other sounds you'll suddenly notice. Bear in mind that you probably lost your hearing over a period of years. You've forgotten that you've ever heard footsteps, sounds of your own chewing and breathing, or water dripping, clocks ticking, and dishes clicking. It's like moving to a new neighborhood: You immediately notice all the new noises.

• Persistence pays. If you take off the aids every time the new sounds become annoying, you'll never adjust. Perhaps the best way to ease yourself into wearing the aids is to set up a schedule. Don't wear the aids home the first day. Take them home in the box, take the aids out in a quiet place, insert them and read out loud. Do that for as long as it's comfortable. Put them in and take them out frequently, adding to your wearing time. Invite one friend over and have some conversation. Then, in a few days, have two friends over. After a few days, you'll be ready to try a walk outside or a drive in the car wearing the aids. Be aware that you will notice a lot of new sounds when driving the car. Many people discover a lot of odd noises coming from their car. One gentleman found that the repairs that his car needed—now that he could hear the car malfunctioning—cost more than the aids.

So, what you've done is to gradually increase your wearing time. Try to do this over at least five days.

• Use of hearing aids can cause moisture to build up in the ear canal, wax glands to block, and skin to become compressed and irritated. This can lead to eczema (dermatitis) with scaling and discomfort. See your doctor for treatment who will probably prescribe cortisone cream.

Maintanence of Hearing Aids

It's a good idea to periodically check your hearing aids. Here's what to look for:

✓ Wax in the sound opening or vent holes

✓ Cracks or separations in the case or tubing on BTE aids

✓ Smooth rotation of the volume wheel with a gradual increase in volume as it turns and no static

✓ Any distortion when saying six sounds that cover the speech range: e (as in beet), o (as in show), u (as in boot), s, sh, m

✓ Clear switches and microphone openings of any debris

Even though you run through these checks faithfully, an aid probably will need repair from time to time. But you can cut your trips to the dispenser by doing your own troubleshooting. Often the problem is minor. This troubleshooting chart will help you recognize and correct some of the more common simple problems.

Hearing Aid Troubleshooting

Problem	What to do
Aid does not work at all	Try a new battery. (The procedure for inserting a battery should have been explained by the person who sold you the aid. If not, get an explanation now, or check the instructions that came with the aid.) Check to make sure that the battery is not reversed (with the plus and minus sides facing in the wrong direction). Usually the battery door won't close if the battery is in backwards. Inspect the tubing on BTE's to insure that it is not bent and crimping off the sound. Make certain that the BTE earmold or the ITE/ITC canal is not plugged with wax. If the hearing aid has a T–switch for telephone use (more on this in Chapter 10) make sure it is not in the T position. Still not working? Call the dispenser.
Aid is working but weak	Replace the battery. Batteries give full output until the last few hours of life. As soon as the battery starts to weaken, throw it away.

Aid is working but weak (cont.)	Make sure that the earmold is inserted properly. Your ear canal may be plugged with wax. A doctor can easily check it out.
Aid gives inter-mit-tent or scratchy signals	The on-off switch may be dusty where it makes electrical contact inside the aid. Turn the switch on and off several times or rotate the volume wheel. If it's a body aid, check the cords for crimping or fraying. If it still gives an intermittent or scratchy signal, the aid needs repair.
Aid makes whistling or squealing sound	The hearing aid is feeding back, just as a loud–speaker feeds back if a microphone is too close. The sound of the loudspeaker is picked up by the microphone, amplified by the speaker, picked up again by the microphone, amplified again, and so on, until the sound has been ampli-fied to a loud howl. To find out why an ITE or ITC is squealing, cover up the hole that goes into the ear and also cover up the vent hole. Turn the aid up as high as possible. If it still squeals with these holes covered, there is an electrical malfunction and the unit needs to be repaired. If the squeal does not occur when you run this test, but does occur when the aid is in your ear, it either does not fit cor-rectly—meaning you'll need another

Aid makes
whistling or
squealing sound
(cont.)

fitting by the dispenser—or the aid is not seated properly.

To find out why a behind-the-ear aid is feeding back, first take the aid off and cover up any opening in the earmold (including the tiny vent holes that are sometimes drilled) and see if the feedback stops. If it does stop, the earmold may not have been correctly inserted, or else it does not fit your ear properly. See your dispenser for instructions again on how to insert it properly, or for another earmold.

If it still squeals, take off the tubing and earmold. Place your finger over the end of the hearing aid that the tubing fits on (the hook). If the squealing stops, the tubing is probably cracked, or does not fit properly into the earmold. See your dispenser for repair.

If the squealing continues, there is probably some internal damage, and the aid needs repair.

One other situation can cause an ITE or ITC aid to squeal: If you have an aid with an extremely large vent, the aid may squeal when you bring your hand near it. If this happens, use just your finger to adjust the volume; point your finger and keep the rest of your hand as far away from your ear as possible. Sometimes feedback is tough to stop because your jaw movement

Aid makes whistling or squealing sound (cont.)

expands the ear canal and breaks the acoustic seal with the aid. So, if all else fails to stop the feedback at comfortable loudness levels, ask your dispenser about "soft wraps" from Comply which wrap around the end of the aid in your ear canal to stop the leak causing feedback and keep a loose aid in the ear.

And last, an ear canal full of wax will reflect sound back and cause feedback.

Aid using up batteries too quickly

Battery life is determined by the power of the aid and the type of battery, and can be anywhere from 50 to 1,000 hours of use—when the hearing aid is actually on. The average battery life is probably close to 150–300 hours. The hearing aid dispenser can give you an estimate of battery life based on your particular aid and the brand of batteries you use. You should keep a diary of the number of hours the aid is in use; the time may be much longer than you realize.

Maybe you are buying too many batteries at a time or from a place that keeps them on the shelf for a long time. (The term "shelf life" is used to refer to battery life in an unopened package.) Zinc batteries start to discharge once the tab on the back of the aid is removed. Putting the tab back on will not help much. They will only last about six

Aid using up batteries too quickly (Cont.)	weeks even if you don't use them in the aid. One package, usually 4, 8, or 10 batteries, should last you a reasonable amount of time. Hearing aid dispensers are the most likely place to have the freshest batteries. If you still feel the batteries are being used up too quickly, check to see if you may accidentally be leaving the aid turned on at night. Are batteries still draining too quickly? There may be an electronic problem, so take the aid for repair.
Aid produces distorted, unclear signal	Change the battery. Some aids are distorted or produce a motorboat–like sound in the last minutes of battery life. Check for earwax plugging up the opening. If neither of these steps help, the unit needs professional repair.
Moisture collects in the tubing of the BTE aid	This is common. As the warm air from the inside of your ear goes into the cooler tubing the water vapor will condense and collect on the tubing. This will usually not cause a problem unless there is a great deal of moisture, in which case the tubing can become plugged. You can buy a small dehumidifier pack from your dealer to store your aid in at night. This will reduce the moisture, but you'll have to have the tubing changed more frequently because it will dry out sooner. Even ITE/ITC aids will be affected by constant

Moisture collects in the tubing of the BTE aid (Cont.)	humidity and may need a dehumidifier pack.

Difficulties with hearing aids don't always, of course, stem from trouble with the instrument itself. The batteries are often the source of the problem. It is critical that you use the correct size and type of battery, or the aid will not work properly.

The type of battery in popular use is called a zinc or zinc air battery. Previously mercury batteries were common, but state governments are outlawing them because of environmental pollution. And (expensive) silver oxide batteries are rarely used now even for power aids. Zinc batteries expose zinc to air through holes in the outside of the battery; the interaction of zinc and air produces the electrical current. Zinc batteries will come with a plastic tab on the back to keep air out and the battery fresh until you use the battery.

How long does a battery last? That's difficult to predict, because it depends on the size of the battery, the power and circuitry in the hearing aid, how long the aid is worn, and how loudly it is turned up when used. But to give a ballpark figure, you can usually expect a zinc battery to last about 300 hours with analog aids.

As mentioned, the size of the battery also has an impact on its useful life. Most hearing aid batteries come in one of four sizes. Size 675 (the numbers are arbitrary—they don't mean anything in and of themselves) is a little smaller than a dime. It looks like a standard wristwatch battery but it's not—don't try to use a wristwatch battery in your hearing aid. The 675 battery is most often used in behind-the-ear models.

The next size down is size 13. This is usually used for small behind-the-ear and many in-the-ear aids.

Some small in-the-ear and most in-the-canal aids use

a battery called size 312. The very tiny in-the-canal aids may use either a 230 or size 10. (Both numbers refer to the same size battery.)

Check with your dispenser to make sure you know the proper size battery for your aid. The brand name (the maker) is not important but the size definitely is. You can and probably will damage your aid if you try to insert the wrong size battery.

You can buy batteries from your hearing aid dispenser, in drug stores, and electronics supply stores. If you are a member of the American Association of Retired Persons (AARP) check their literature for sales on hearing aid batteries. Regardless of where you buy them, be sure that the batteries are fresh. Check the date on the package to make sure they are not expired.

You should be aware of some special notes on batteries:

- It's a good idea to open the battery drawer at night. This makes doubly sure that the aid is off, and also allows the battery and its compartment to dry out. Moisture deteriorates hearing aids.
- Don't bother trying to squeeze a few extra hours out of a battery that is going bad and producing a weak, distorted, or motor–boat–like sound. Batteries go dead very quickly, so you're not gaining much by suffering with a dying battery.
- Don't carry batteries loose in your pocket, especially with coins. Contact with the change in your pocket or purse can discharge the batteries. Use the carrying case in which your batteries came, or get a special carrying case from your dealer.
- Be careful how you dispose of batteries. If swallowed by pets or children (or even an adult with poor eyesight who mistakes it for a pill) they can cause serious internal damage. If one is swallowed,

call this emergency hot line collect: (202) 625–3333 or a physician.

• Once the battery shows signs of weakening, throw it away. Even though it will recover a bit overnight, you'll still only get a few more hours out of it, which will only save you pennies and might get it mixed up with good batteries.

• Turning the aids on and off during the day to save batteries isn't worth it. You might miss something important and it is inconsiderate of others to "turn them off." And again, the few pennies you might save per battery isn't worth it.

Common Problems

The new experience of wearing an aid can be difficult to cope with. There may be no simple solution; however, an understanding of why the situation annoys you may help you deal with the problem. Here are some of the more common difficulties.

Hearing Aid User Complaints

Problem	Explanation
When I work in the kitchen, the sound of dishes clinking together drives me crazy.	You are bothered by sudden high–frequency sounds, such as dishes clinking. It is probably quite annoying because you haven't heard these sounds in a while, or you have only heard the low frequencies in these sounds. In some cases, a condition called recruitment (an abnormal sensitivity to loudness) will cause sudden, high–frequency sounds to be uncomfortable. You may soon adjust to the new sounds coming through the hearing aid, though. If

you can't get used to them, the hearing aid dispenser may adjust the aid.

I Hate the unnatural sound of the hearing aid.

Since you have a hearing loss, "natural" for you means not hearing well. As mentioned earlier in the chapter, the hearing aid must change the nature of sound; the change, while less natural–sounding, will allow better hearing. Most hearing aid users become accustomed to this different type of sound. If you don't become used to the new sound in two or more weeks, take the aid back to the dispenser for adjustment.

I get so much wax in my ears now that I wear a hearing aid.

The presence of the earmold or the aid may stimulate wax production. People who don't wear hearing aids get wax in their ears, too, but it gradually falls out of the ear canal. With an earmold or aid in place, much of the wax is retained. You may have to visit a physician from time to time and have the wax removed; this is a simple and painless procedure. Be sure to ask your hearing aid dispenser for a system to keep the wax from getting inside the hearing aids.

The ear piece hurts.

In the beginning, the ear piece may be slightly uncomfortable, but it shouldn't cause soreness, redness, or irritation. It's much like wearing a new pair of shoes, and you will probably soon become used to it. However, if the ear piece still is uncomfortable after a few days, or if you notice irritated spots in your ear, go back to the dispenser and have it altered. It's also possible to be allergic to the material in hearing aids or earmolds. If so, the skin in contact with the aid will change color, weep and/or itch like crazy. It may even swell. There are hypoallergenic materials available. Ask your dispenser.

Everything is so loud! I can't stand it!

When you're coming out of a movie theater into bright sunshine, the light hurts your eyes. Much the same situation occurs when you have become used to a hearing loss and suddenly put on an aid. It may take days or weeks for you to adjust to your new–found hearing when you first get an aid. If you still are bothered after three or four weeks, or if it is actually painful to wear the aid at any time, return to the dispenser. Having the characteristics of the aid re-adjusted may allow a compromise between good hearing and tolerance of the sound.

I wore my new hearing aids to a meeting yesterday and it was unbearable.

Hearing aids take getting used to, and a room full of people is not the place to start. Begin by wearing the aids alone in a quiet room, and read aloud. After you've become used to the sound of your own voice, invite another person in to speak with you. Gradually increase the number of people in the communication situation; you may also want to experiment with various levels of background noise to simulate real–world conditions. Putting on the aid and immediately venturing into a difficult communication situation can quickly alienate a new wearer; this is one reason why so many aids wind up in the drawer after only one use. You will probably want to allow three or four weeks before you are wearing the aid full time in all types of situations.

My own voice sounds strange.

This is normal because you are not used to hearing yourself as others hear you. Remember the first time you heard yourself on a tape recorder? You will adjust to the "new voice" within a few days. But if your voice continues to sound hollow or it echoes (or you have a "full" feeling in your ear) report this problem to your hearing aid dispenser, who can adjust the aid and/or your earmold.

While your own voice may seem loud at first, it is important to remember that you should adjust the hearing aid for other people's voices, not your own. Once you hear others at the correct level, your voice will automatically adjust itself.

Incidentally, never forget that when you pay for an aid, you are paying for services including counseling and adjustment. Be an assertive consumer. Your dispenser will almost always rather have you bring your problems directly to him or her, rather than have you tell others of your dissatisfaction.

It is very important that you talk to your hearing aid dispenser about problems with your aids. If (s)he doesn't know about a problem, it can't be fixed. But you must make your comments useful. Telling your doctor that "your head hurts" isn't useful. Describing the pain as sharp, dull, or throbbing, locating where it is in the head, and reporting when and how often it occurs, is useful. Telling your dispenser, "my aid whistles" needs to be followed by information on when, at what volume level, and in what environments. "It doesn't help in noisy places" is more useful if you include whether the loudness of the noise is intolerable, or you just can't understand speech. Just saying that "it doesn't sound natural" needs to be clarified with a description such as muffled, tinny, soft, static, etc.

If you've never worn hearing aids, and are considering getting them, knowing about these typical problems beforehand will, at least, let you know that you're not alone. All the problems haven't been covered, of course; it's evident just from the length of this chapter how broad the topic is. Related information will be presented in later chapters: how an audiologist (Chapter 8) selects the right kind of hearing aids, and how to deal with the people who sell hearing aids (Chapter 9). You should see a physician before getting aids, and that will be the subject of the next chapter. First, here are some of the more common questions asked about hearing aids:

What brand of hearing aid should I buy?
You are best off if you stick to a major brand, but no one brand is best for everybody. It is not the brand,

but the particular model, that is important. Different types of hearing losses require various hearing aid models; if a particular brand is recommended to you it is probably because that manufacturer makes a model with characteristics that fit your hearing loss. But it does not mean that the particular manufacturer is the only one who makes the right type of aid. A listing of major hearing aid brands is included in Chapter 9.

Incidentally, it's important to point out that what you really want to shop for is the dispenser, not the brand. There are no brands that are best for everybody, but there are clearly superior dispensers. Ask your friends with hearing aids for their recommendations.

I know that you have used "style" to describe the way a hearing aid is worn, that is, behind-the-ear, in-the-ear, and so on. And I know what "brand" means. But then what do you mean by "model"?

Model refers to the characteristics that are built into a hearing aid, determining the quantity and quality of sound that the hearing aid can provide. As noted above, different types of hearing losses require different combinations of these characteristics. Each particular combination that a manufacturer makes is called a model. A large hearing aid manufacturer, for example, might make twenty different models of aids, each of which is designed to fit the needs of a particular hearing loss. However, the flexibility of digital components is reducing the number of models needed.

The four major characteristics are:

1. *Gain*—the power of the instrument, how much it amplifies sound. The greater your hearing loss, the more gain you'll probably need.

2. *Frequency range*—how much power there is in

certain pitch ranges, and how far the amplification ability of the aid extends into the high and low pitches. If, for example, you have a loss in the high pitches (perhaps because of many years of exposure to loud noise) you will need an aid designed to boost high frequencies.

3. *Maximum power output*—the loudest sound the aid will produce, regardless of how much sound is put into it. This characteristic insures comfort, and acts as a safeguard against damage to the ears.

4. *Distortion*—a measure of how faithfully the hearing aid reproduces the sound that comes into it. Any electronic instrument, including your television, for example, distorts the sound signal to some extent, which is why you may have trouble understanding actors and speakers. There is a triple distortion: the television, your impaired hearing mechanism, and the hearing aid itself. On top of all that, you really can't read lips on television, and it's hard to pick up other cues that would help you to understand.

I notice many of my friends wearing two hearing aids. Why is that?

Good question. There are many advantages to wearing binaural (two) aids, and the practice has recently become much more popular. About 65 percent of users wear two hearing aids now. Although wearing two aids can be more bothersome and will be more expensive, you'll benefit from not having a "bad side." You will feel more oriented or balanced in space with two aids. Having two ears to listen with helps you to localize sound much more easily, so you'll spend less time spinning your head around, trying to figure out who is talking to you among a group of people; this is extremely helpful if you are lipreading, and need to pick up on conversation quickly. There's another advantage, too: background noise can be less troublesome when you are listening with two ears. Since you probably don't hear well in noise at any time, have a friend with normal hearing try this experiment to prove it: listen to someone speak in background noise. Then plug one ear tightly and carry on the conversation. The noise will seem much more distracting and the person's voice will blend in with the noise when the ear is plugged. Unplug the ear and the voice will seem to pop out from the noise.

Another advantage to wearing two aids is that neither of the aids has to be turned up as loudly as when wearing only one. This helps tolerate background noise, reduces feedback, and aids overall comfort. But probably the biggest advantage to wearing two aids is that you will hear better, even in quiet situations. There is more information going to your brain so it is easier to figure out the message.

If it is financially feasible, two aids are almost always better than one. While binaural aids are less successful for people with a large difference in the hearing loss of one ear compared to the other, sometimes even this difficult-to-fit group can benefit from two aids. People with slight or very severe hearing losses, or those with only basic communication requirements, may also find less benefit from two aids.

By the way, you may as well try two aids. Dispensers should sell aids with a thirty-day money-back guarantee. If you find you get along well with just one aid, you can return the other. But be sure to get used to the two aids for at least two-to-three weeks before you start taking one off to compare the effect.

One other point: You don't always have to wear

two aids. You can, for example, wear one aid when you are alone at home. Once you get used to two aids though, you will probably feel most comfortable with both of them all the time.

A final point. Recent research is discovering that "if you don't use it, you lose it." In other words, if you have a hearing loss in both ears, and you only get one hearing aid, for some people the unaided ear weakens over the years in its ability to process (understand) speech. So the use of a second aid in the previously unaided ear years later may not be successful because it sounds distorted. It may actually interfere with the clearer sound in your other ear. With long term practice, you may recover some of this ability. Incidentally, the same thing can happen if you have a high-pitched hearing loss in both ears for a long time. Since your brain is not getting any high-pitched information, it just assigns the high pitch portion of itself to another function. The addition of high pitches through a hearing aid at a later date may not be helpful in understanding speech because the brain has been altered to function without them.

On the other hand, a few older people actually do better with one aid. They report too much confusion of sounds with two aids and prefer one. But the only way to determine if you are one of these people is to get two aids and give them a fair trial first.

Do I have to wear the hearing aids all the time?

For the first eight weeks you should wear the aids at least six to eight hours a day to practice using them in different situations. After you develop good judgment about the benefits of the aids, you can wear them whenever they help you. You'll probably want to wear them most of the time to get full benefit. Asking your brain to keep adjusting to two different listening systems (aided and unaided) all the time isn't good.

I feel embarrassed about wearing the aids. When will I get over it?

Probably as soon as you fully realize all the benefits of wearing the aids. For some people, embarrassment is a natural reaction, but remember that a hearing aid is much less visible than you probably think it is. Besides, by wearing the aids you can save yourself a lot of embarrassment that stems from mistakes in conversation. Your hearing loss is more conspicuous than hearing aids.

Aids are not unusual items anymore. You see them everywhere. Once you start telling people about your loss and the hearing aids, you'll be surprised how easy it is. If you try to hide it, people will think there is a problem. If you are open about it, they will see there is a solution to a problem.

I don't have hearing aids at the present time. How do I tell when I really need them?

You need aids when you are having significant difficulty in communication, and a physician has told you that there is no medical help. If you are not hearing things that you need to, or want to, you are probably a good candidate. An audiologist can confirm your suspicions, but can not tell whether you are having problems—only you can tell that for sure. Don't be satisfied with just "getting along OK." It is much better to be "doing well." Different people in different situations will vary in their need for a hearing aid. A retired person who lives alone will have very different needs than a librarian, who constantly deals with people who are speaking softly.

In summary, there is no magical formula. Your need for hearing aids depends on a combination of lifestyle, degree of hearing loss, age, and motivation. Only you can determine how lifestyle, age and motivation factor in. That's a question you—not your doctor or audiologist—must answer. But be sure your answer is an honest one. You are only deceiving yourself if you prevaricate.

Is there any hearing aid that does not have anything that goes inside the ear?

Yes, there is; it's called a bone conduction aid and is rarely used for people who have a conductive hearing loss. The aid is really a vibrator on a headband usually worn against the bone in back of the ear. This system vibrates the bones of the skull, bypassing the inadequate outer or middle ear, and sends the sound directly to the inner ear (which would for this application, be normal).

These aids are bulky, uncomfortable at times, and do not provide a very clear sound. They are rarely used today because the other types of aids, described previously, are better. There are also the implantable aids described earlier. But these are a rather drastic solution. If anatomy allows, give the ones inside the ear a chance.

I've heard about rechargeable hearing aids. Do they work?

Yes, but with limitations. The primary drawback is that if you forget to plug in the charging unit, you're out a hearing aid until it recharges. Secondly, the rechargeable units have to be changed periodically, about once a year, and that may cost more than the batteries.

There is even a solar powered aid which has come out, but hasn't seemed to catch on, so there must be some problems with the device.

What about the hearing aids advertised on TV and in magazines?

Remember that if it sounds too good to be true, it probably is. With those low cost hearing aids or "amplifiers" you usually get what you pay for. Remember that hearing aids are complex electronic instruments that require personal fitting and knowledgeable adjustments by a qualified person. Beware of high pressure sales techniques, visits to your home, anything free, or phrases like "for nerve losses" (most aids are for that) or "eliminates noise."

How loud should the hearing aid be?

Some dispensers will tell you a specific volume range, which is most helpful if you have a dial with numbers on it. It's probably better to set the aid by instinct. Remember, if it's too low, the hearing aid will act as a plug and actually obstruct your hearing. If set too high, the aid will cause discomfort and distortion. One of the better ways to set the volume is to turn it up until it reaches the level of discomfort, then back off slightly. Don't set the volume just below the sound of feedback. That may be too soft for optimum hearing. If it squeals at comfortable levels, talk to your dispenser. With some of the new technology, the compression circuit does the work for you and you don't even need a volume wheel.

My hearing loss is only in the high pitches. I've been told that a hearing aid will not help. True?

Probably not. Recent advances in technology have allowed us to amplify very high pitches while not significantly boosting lower pitches. As you remember, it is the high pitches that lend speech its intelligibility. Interestingly, some people with essentially normal hearing sensitivity on a hearing test find that they like wearing an aid to make listening to speech more comfortable. The hearing aids may become an instrument of convenience as well as necessity, similar to reading glasses used by people with basically adequate vision.

However, once a hearing loss in the high pitches reaches a certain degree of severity (about 60 dB), amplifying that region does not seem to help in understanding speech. In that event, there is new technology being developed which actually shifts the sound of people's voices to a lower pitch—it's called frequency transposition or compression. Thus, those with high frequency losses can understand speech better by hearing it in the lower pitches.

I understand that there are hearing aids that use no battery. Do they work?

Not very well. They're essentially an "ear trumpet" that helps sound resonate better. They have met with limited success and are only for very mild hearing losses. Cupping your hand behind your ear causes a 15 db gain at about 2000 Hz, which is similar to these instruments. It helps, but not enough for most losses or most situations.

Will my hearing get worse if I wear aids?

No, but after hearing better for a while, your unaided condition will just seem worse in comparison.

My mom is in a nursing home and I worry about whether she gets full use of the hearing aids I bought her. What should I ask?

If your mom can't handle the aids herself, find out who puts the aids on and off for her. Do they also adjust the volume if necessary? Who changes the batteries? Does anyone check for impacted earwax? Does she get periodic hearing tests? Do they just turn the aids down if they whistle? Does anyone routinely check eyeglasses and hearing aids to be certain they're functioning? Is there a system to be sure the aids don't get lost, like a retention-clip that secures the aids to her clothing?

What does the future hold in hearing aids?

That is pretty tough to predict, but here are a few possibilities:

• Disposable aids have already been developed by some prominent scientists and engineers at Songbird Medical Inc. These will be about $40 and will last 30-45 days before the battery gives out and the whole thing is disposed of. No impression of the ear is required. The early ones are available now, but look for others to follow soon. Note that these will probably have a limited application to mild high frequency hearing losses and should be fitted by a licensed dispenser after an evaluation.

• Virtual test environments will allow us to try out hearing aids ahead of time under many different conditions.

• Beam forming arrays of microphones, maybe in eyeglasses or necklaces, will allow hearing in noise even better than normal hearing.

• Application of cochlear implants to those with much less a degree of hearing loss.

• And in the far future, maybe even hair cell regeneration and gene therapy to "cure" losses so we won't need hearing aids.

{ 7 }
The Physician

Once you've made the decision to get a hearing aid, you must eventually be seen by a physician. In fact, according to a regulation of the Food and Drug Administration, the hearing aid dispenser is not supposed to sell you a hearing aid until you have done so. Before you buy the aid, you must produce a note from the doctor, certifying that there is no medical reason why you should not have a hearing aid. There are several good reasons for this:

- Before the federal regulation concerning the visit to the doctor, some people were being sold hearing aids when there was a medical or surgical technique that could restore some or all of their hearing.
- In unusual cases, a hearing loss can be the symptom of a serious medical problem. For example, a hearing loss can be caused by diabetes, a thyroid condition, a kidney problem, or a tumor on the auditory nerve.
- There are certain medical conditions that can be aggravated by a hearing aid, such as an ear infection.

There is currently a movement to have this regulation modified because of the increased monitoring of who can sell hearing aids. When the regulation was passed, many states had no restriction on who could sell aids. However, now that most states have some form of hearing aid dispenser licensure or regulation, those who fit aids should have had training and passed an exam which would include appropriate referral to physicians when needed. By-passing the physician visit would eliminate an extra cost for those who have a straight age related or noise induced loss and do not need medical help. But don't make the decision to by-pass a physician by yourself.

A physician who specializes in diseases of the ear should be able to spot any of these situations where a hearing aid is not appropriate, although the clearance you need can be obtained from any type of medical doctor. The regulation was written this way because specialists are hard to find in some remote areas of the country. However, you should visit a specialist if at all possible.

The kind of doctor you want to see is usually called an ear, nose, and throat doctor, or ENT. An ENT is a physician who has earned a medical degree and then undertaken extra study in the ear, nose, and throat field, combined with a residency at a hospital. ENT physicians are also known as head and neck surgeons or as *otorhinolaryngologists* (*oto* means ear, *rhino* indicates nose, and *laryngo* stands for throat). ENT means the same thing, and is a lot easier to say. Some of these specialists limit their practice entirely to ears and call themselves *otologists*.

Does this mean that an ENT or otologist will be an expert on hearing aids and other aspects of coping with hearing loss? No, it does not: While these physicians are highly trained in the pathology of the ear, and possess great skill in medical and surgical procedures, they may not be well versed in the problems caused by a communication handicap and the rehabilitative procedures available. Some ENTs take a personal interest in communication problems, but with the staggering amount of research they must keep up with, it's next to impossible for these specialists to be aware of all the developments in the field of *aural rehabilitation* (therapy and devices to help a hearing impaired person communicate better).

This essentially means that it will be your responsibility to make sure you're getting an informed opinion on the topic of hearing aids and communication problems. Don't be afraid to question your doctor, to discuss your communication problems, or to ask for a referral to someone who might be more adept in these matters. Just assure the doctor that you are aware of his expertise in medical matters and you can't expect him to keep up on the communicative aspect of your problem. First, though, be satisfied that there is nothing that can be done medically or surgically to alleviate your hearing loss.

If, for example, you suffer from otosclerosis (where the tiny sound–conducting bones in the middle ear lose their ability to vibrate), surgery may help to restore hearing. Also, most hearing losses that result from middle ear infections can be treated medically or surgically. A general rule of thumb states that if the problem is centered in the outer or middle ear, there's a chance that it may be cured. If the loss is secondary to another condition such as poor circulation, an infection, a metabolic imbalance, or a tumor, medical treatment is indicated for the primary problem.

Inner-ear hearing losses rarely respond to any sort of treatment. However, there have been cases where a loss is caused by a medical ailment such as high cholesterol or renal disease and control of the disease has improved hearing somewhat. The damage from noise exposure or normal deterioration is irreversible. If the hearing loss results from deterioration of nerve pathways up to the brain, it's permanent. *Only a physician can tell for sure if medical or surgical intervention can help your particular case.*

What will happen when you visit the doctor for the medical examination that is needed before you can buy hearing aids? First, the doctor will probably take an extensive case history of your problem, and then look in your ears with an otoscope, the familiar flashlight device found in most doctors' offices. The ENT will be looking for any obvious problem with the ear canal or eardrum.

The next step may involve tests for balance and coordination; these are done to see if the hearing loss might stem from a neurological problem. The doctor may also use a tuning fork to make a rough estimate of how well you can hear the sound it gives off.

Following the examination, the doctor may recommend an evaluation by an audiologist (next chapter) or other tests, depending on what was found during the examination. Often, you may be asked to return after these tests are carried out. ENTs sometimes have an audiologist on staff who may do the hearing test during your visit. In either case, there will be an extra charge for the test.

Eventually, the doctor will give you a diagnosis and recommendations; this is when problems can arise. Doctors may be in a hurry and anxious to move on to other scheduled patients. As a result, they sometimes give instructions rather than explanations. It is very important that you ask questions at this point and insist on a complete explanation of your problem. If you don't understand, ask the doctor to restate it in simpler terms. What the doctor says will be very important to you, and since you are paying for it, *you have a right to a thorough explanation, as well as a discussion of all your alternatives.*

Don't accept a physician's statement that you don't have a hearing loss—if you think you do—or you have a hearing loss but nothing can be done for you. That probably means that there are no medical or surgical techniques to cure your loss. There is help for you in the non-medical realm. Insist on seeing an audiologist. Don't accept a statement that you can't use hearing aids because you have nerve deafness, severely reduced speech-understanding ability, good hearing in the low pitches, or a loss only in one ear. Nerve deafness just means you have a sensori-neural hearing loss, the kind being fitted with aids for the past 40-50 years. And all of those other conditions can be accommodated with modern hearing aids.

Here are some questions you might want to ask. If you think you may get flustered and forget, take this list with you.

Questions to Ask Your Doctor

• Is there anything that can be done to alleviate my hearing loss?
• Will it be permanent?
• Is there something that can be done medically or surgically? If there is, will I have a residual hearing loss after treatment?
• If surgery is recommended; is it necessary for my health? Can I get along without surgery? (Some people have hearing loss that could be corrected surgically, but, for their own reasons, choose not to have surgery and to wear hearing aids. This is all right unless the condition causing the hearing loss endangers health.)
• Can you refer me to a good audiologist, one who is particularly interested in hearing aids and aural rehabilitation? (Some audiologists are more interested in other aspects of hearing loss, such as diagnosis of particular disorders, educational audiology for children, or academic research.)
• How much will all this cost me? How much is the

office visit? The hearing test? Any further treatment or tests? (Don't feel as though you're being stingy, by the way. Remember that the richest people in the world got their money that way.)
• What part of my treatment, if any, is covered by Medicare, Medicaid, or other insurance? (More on this in Chapter 14.)
• Do you think I might benefit from hearing aids? If not, why?

There may be times when you want a second opinion—especially if surgery is indicated. Admittedly, it's a bother and an additional expense to see another doctor, but you must weigh that against the cost and risk of surgery. Even if no surgery or medical treatment is recommended, you may feel as though your doctor doesn't know or care about your particular problem. Don't ever feel bad about getting a second opinion. Doctors are fallible, and don't have all the answers.

The next chapter will explain the procedures used by audiologists. First, questions on dealing with physicians:

What right do I have to disagree with my doctor? I don't have a medical degree.

If you disagree about whether your hearing loss causes a communication problem, you have every right in the world to differ with your doctor. After all, it is your problem, and in that sense you know more about it than anyone else in the world.

Are any of the doctor's tests painful?

Not really. The only discomfort you may feel would result from a specialized test called electronystagmography, which often makes people dizzy and nauseated. This test is only done in cases where certain inner-ear problems are suspected. Removal of earwax can be a bit uncomfortable if it is impacted or hardened. You can ask to come back for the removal after putting a softening agent in your ear.

Doctors are so expensive. Is there any way I can save money?
If a hearing loss is your only concern, you can check to see if you really do have a significant hearing loss before you see a doctor. In many places, hearing screenings are offered free or at reduced cost. Check at colleges, health fairs, or senior citizen centers. The result of the hearing screening will tell you whether to pursue the matter and see a doctor or audiologist.

Suppose I want hearing aids but don't want to see a doctor?
The federal regulation allows you to sign a waiver if it is against your personal beliefs to see a doctor; the waiver states that even though you understand it is in your best interest to see a physician, you choose not to. Even if the federal regulation is modified, audiologists may cover themselves by having a waiver signed anyway. For reasons already explained, using this waiver to skip an examination is not a good idea. Some people who have had hearing aids in the past choose not to see the doctor again, but you should be aware that medical problems can develop within this time. If any of these factors are present, you should definitely see a doctor:
- sudden change in hearing in one or both ears
- drainage/pain/discomfort in the ears
- constant attacks of dizziness
- excessive earwax
- malformation of the ear

What role do diet and health play in hearing loss?

Aging, infection, and noise are not the only causes of acquired hearing losses. Just as with other body organs, the ear can be affected by overall body health. Excessive intake of salt, alcohol, tobacco, and caffeine, as well as vitamin deficiencies, can cause metabolic imbalances that inhibit body function, including hearing.

Conditions such as high cholesterol, diabetes, heart disease, pulmonary, or renal problems can restrict a healthy blood flow to the ears and cause damage.

Meniere disease, where there is too much inner-ear fluid, is thought to be linked to metabolic problems. Some people find relief from the symptoms through decreasing sodium and increasing potassium in their diet, and diuretics may be prescribed by physicians.

Some people have specific food allergies that lead to disorders throughout the body, including the ears.

Shouldn't my family doctor detect a hearing loss?

Maybe, but only about 16% of the overall population, 18% of the 65-74 age group, and 22% of the over age 75 group are routinely screened for hearing loss by their physicians.

So don't depend on them. If you think you have a problem, follow up yourself.

{ 8 }
The Audiologist

It's odd that even though the number of audiologists in the United States is constantly on the increase (about 12,000), many people have little if any idea of what an audiologist is. Because audiologists are your first line of defense in preventing a hearing loss from making your life difficult and souring your emotional outlook, it is important that you understand what audiologists are, what they can do, and how they do it.

An audiologist is a professional trained in the non-medical aspects of hearing impairment, such as evaluation of hearing loss and rehabilitation of the hearing impaired. Audiologists have earned either a master's degree or doctorate, have served an internship, and have passed a qualifying examination. An audiologist can be a fellow of the American Academy of Audiology (FAAA) and/or can have a Certificate of Clinical Competence in Audiology (CCC-A) from the American Speech Language Hearing Association (ASHA). In almost all states they are licensed by a state government licensing board which actually defines their legal right to practice in that state. Most of these credentials require a certain amount of continuing education to keep current. Most audiologists keep these certificates on their office wall.

Along the way, an audiologist learns how speech and hearing develop; how to prevent hearing losses;

how problems arise with hearing; how to test for hearing loss; how various methods of rehabilitation help people with a hearing loss. This type of rehabilitation is called aural rehabilitation, and the basic tools are therapy, counseling, and electronic devices.

Although not all audiologists specialize in the same aspect of hearing loss, they generally provide these services:

- A screening: to determine if someone has a hearing loss significant enough to follow up on.
- A hearing evaluation: a complete set of tests to determine the amount of hearing loss, the type and location of the loss, and the degree of handicap that may result.
- A hearing aid evaluation: to determine the characteristics of the hearing aids that will best suit an individual's hearing loss. In some cases the audiologist will sell hearing aids. Audiologists who have joined this recent trend prefer to call themselves "dispensers" rather than "dealers," a distinction that will be explained in the next chapter. In most cases the audiologist will sell and fit the hearing aids.
- Therapy and counseling: to help the hearing impaired person improve communication and cope with the hearing loss. This is a rapidly growing area of audiology, and will be covered in Chapter 11.

Where do you find an audiologist?

They usually work in a rehabilitation center, a speech and hearing center, a hospital, an ENT'S office, a college or university, or in private practice. They are often listed in the yellow pages. If a college or university in your area trains students in speech and hearing, there is probably a clinic on campus that offers reduced fees because it serves as a training ground for students (who are under the supervision of a fully qualified audiologist).

When calling a college or university, don't ask the person at the switchboard "whether the college gives hearing tests." Switchboard operators may not be completely informed about activities on campus. Instead, ask for the department of communication disorders, speech and hearing (sciences), or speech pathology and audiology. If the operator can't find the first one you ask for, try all three, because the person on the other end of the telephone will probably just be scanning an alphabetical directory, and might not realize that you want *speech pathology* and *audiology* when you've asked for *speech and hearing.*

Once you are connected with the right department, ask to speak to a faculty member, preferably an audiologist, who should be able to tell you about the availability of hearing tests. Don't ask a secretary or clerk; in large universities clerical staffers are rotated frequently and you may be speaking to a newcomer who may not know about all of the department's activities.

When you arrange a hearing test at any of the facilities mentioned above, you will be given an appointment. If you're confronted with a long waiting time (longer than two weeks or so), you might elect to try another audiologist.

What will the hearing test be like?
• You will enter a sound-treated booth—a room specially designed to keep out background noise— and will sit facing a window. The audiologist will be on the other side of the window during the testing. First, though, the audiologist will join you in the room and take a case history. If you cannot hear or understand the questions, it is essential that you

say so. Don't guess and risk giving inappropriate or incomplete answers; the audiologist won't mind a bit if you ask to have words repeated, or spoken more slowly. After all, if you didn't have trouble hearing, you wouldn't be there in the first place.

• After the case history, the audiologist may look in your ears with an otoscope to make sure that there is no obstruction, infection, or other factor to affect the test results.

• Following instructions for the first test, a pair of headphones will probably be placed over your ears, and the door to the booth will be shut (but not locked). The audiologist will be on the other side of the window. There will be a microphone channel open so the audiologist will be able to see and hear you at all times.

• Then, the actual testing will begin. Which tests and in what order will depend on your history and the preference of the audiologist. However, there are a few basic tests which are done on almost everyone unless it is a screening where just a pure tone air conduction test (described below) is done. (Keep in mind that a very mild hearing loss usually can't be detected at an event such as a health fair where there is a lot of background noise.) There are other tests—not described—which may be given based on the results on those listed below.

For each test, you will be given instructions, and although there's really no compelling reason for you to know the purpose of these tests, a description of what will happen may satisfy your curiosity about all the mysterious beeps, soft voices, and other sounds you will hear during the thirty minutes to an hour you spend in a hearing evaluation. Here's what the tests are called and what they measure:

• Pure tone air conduction: this is the basic sensitivity test, used in both a complete evaluation and a screening. During the pure tone air conduction test, a series of tones, like musical notes, will be fed through the headphones. The test will be done on one ear at a time. The audiologist will ask you to respond whenever you hear the tone, either by raising your hand or pushing a button. You should respond even when the tone is very faint. The tones will be given at all different loudness levels and pitches; the purpose of this test is to determine the softest level at which you can hear in all the frequency ranges. If you remember the material in chapter 1, you'll understand that this is a test for sensitivity. Also remember that hearing losses occur at different frequencies, so it is important for the audiologist to determine at which frequencies, or pitches, you hear best.

• Pure tone bone conduction: the headphones will be removed for this test. The audiologist will instead place a tiny vibrator behind an ear or on the forehead. This test proceeds in the same manner as the first test, except that the vibrator bypasses the outer and middle ear and directly measures the sensitivity of the inner ear mechanism. Thus, this measures how much of your loss is due to the outer/middle ear and how much is due to the inner ear.

• Impedance/admittance measurements or tympanometry: bone conduction pure tone and this test measure similar things, so results on one may make the other inappropriate. This tests middle ear function and involves bouncing a sound wave off the eardrum and analyzing the return wave. In this procedure, the audiologist does all the work. All you do is sit quietly while the audiologist rather firmly inserts something like an earplug with a wire on the end. This may be slightly uncomfortable, but not painful. You will feel some pressure changes and hear some loud sounds.

• Speech reception or recognition threshold testing: the headphones will be placed back over your ears and the audiologist, through a microphone, will read a list of two-syllable words, such as baseball, cowboy, railroad, and sunset. You are to repeat what was said—there is a microphone in your chamber—or what you think was said. The words will get progressively fainter, and it is important that you take your best guess if you aren't sure of the word spoken. This test will identify how sensitive your ears are to speech.

• Comfortable loudness levels: the audiologist will ask you to make judgements on what is the most comfortable level of loudness, and possibly also the level at which loudness becomes uncomfortable. She will probably just talk to you, adjusting the loudness gradually until you say it is comfortable or uncomfortable, giving you the other options of too loud or too soft to listen to over a long period of time. This will be done a few times to verify it. Remember, what is wanted is the *most* comfortable, so don't just say everything is okay; pick the best level.

• Speech discrimination or word recognition testing (same test, different name): this will measure your ability to understand speech once it's loud enough for you. The audiologist will present a list of 25-50 one syllable words for each ear at a comfortable loudness level. Sometimes the words will be read aloud and sometimes it will be on a recording. You will be asked, for example, to "say the word fail". The words can be very difficult to recognize—you might mistake *fail* for *sail*—so don't become frustrated. You are expected to make some mistakes.

• Masking: you may also, at any time during these tests, hear a sound like waterfall or static in the ear that is not being tested. This noise blocks out that ear to make sure that you're not picking up sound where you are not supposed to.

• Following the hearing evaluation the audiologist will discuss the results, telling you if you have a hearing loss; in which ear(s); how severe it is; what type of loss; where the problem is in your system; and how it affects your communication. If any of these areas are not covered, or if the information is too technical or confusing, stop the person and ask questions. Yes, they may be on a time schedule, but they are also being paid by you or your insurer for service. You have a right to know. If you have a loss, recommendations will be made and will usually include one or more of these (and possibly some others not mentioned):

- go back to a physician for medical examination and possible treatment or for medical clearance to get hearing aids
- come back for a re-test periodically to determine the stability of your hearing loss
- referral to a therapy program to learn better communication techniques
- referral to a support group
- purchase of assistive devices
- purchase of hearing aids

Again, ask for these to be summarized or written down for you at the end of the session, unless you will be getting a copy of the audiology report.

• If hearing aids are indicated, and you have already seen a physician about your loss, the fitting process could start immediately. However, if that audiologist does not dispense aids, or if you want to go elsewhere to get the aids, or if you just need time to get used to the idea, another appointment can be made for the fitting process. Unless you have a definite reason against it, it is usually a good idea to stay with the same audiologist for the hearing aid fitting.

At some point you should be given the opportunity to discuss different styles of hearing aids and various technologies with the audiologist. The advantages and limitations of each, as they relate to your personal needs, should be considered. If the audiologist feels that one style or type of aid is particularly appropriate, you can ask for the reasons why.

You're now ready to purchase hearing aids, the topic of the next chapter. First, let's consider some of the more frequently asked questions about audiologists and hearing tests.

How much does an audiologist charge?
The prices will vary widely, but you can probably expect to pay from $75-125 for a complete hearing evaluation at a clinic or doctor's office unless your health insurance will pay for it. Prices will be lower at a college or university clinic. If you go to a hearing aid dispenser, the initial hearing test is often included in the cost of the hearing aids.

If I go to a clinic at a college or university, won't I be taking a chance by letting students test me?
Students in these clinics are under the direct supervision of a fully qualified (and at many institutions, exceptionally qualified) audiologist. As a matter of fact, the audiologist responsible for the students may be paying closer attention to the tests than if

they were doing them themselves. All results and recommendations will, of course, be reviewed by the supervising audiologist. There is one drawback: Students need more time to conduct the tests, and you occasionally may have to sit around and wait awhile, when something is being explained to them. But because the cost will be lower than if you were tested in a hospital or at a private practice, it may be worth it to you.

The audiologist I'm seeing is called Dr. Robinson. Audiologists aren't doctors, are they?

They are not medical doctors, but some audiologists—usually those in private practice or at universities—have a doctorate in audiology. This degree is earned after about three to five years of additional study beyond the master's degree or four to five years beyond a bachelor's degree. In fact, by the year 2007, the doctoral degree will be the entry level for audiologists. So more and more audiologists will have an Au.D. after their name (clinical doctorate in audiology). Others will have a Ph.D. or an Ed.D., both of which are research doctorates, but most have been trained clinically as well.

How do the results of my tests get to my doctor and hearing aid dispenser?

Part of the audiologist's service involves writing reports and forwarding them to your doctor. You can request a copy of the report if you like, although it is written in technical language and may be hard to understand. You will probably get your hearing aids from the audiologist who does the hearing test, but if not, the hearing aid prescription is usually given to you so you can contact whichever dispensers you wish.

{ 9 }
The Hearing Aid Dispenser

You've probably been wondering when this book would get around to explaining the distinction between a hearing aid "dispenser" and a hearing aid "dealer." The terms have been used interchangeably so far, and you may be somewhat confused—but since the terms actually have no strict definition, it's hard to say when one or the other is correct.

Both refer to someone who sells hearing aids. The primary difference between a hearing aid dispenser and a hearing aid dealer is basically the same as the difference between a *trailer* and a *mobile home*, or an *undertaker* and a *funeral director*. One phrase sounds better than the other, you see, and people concerned with their image have a way of working a more impressive–sounding word into their vocabulary.

When audiologists began to sell hearing aids, they decided that the term *dealer* didn't sound professional enough, and the term *dispenser* was popularized. Recently, the dealers began to express a marked preference toward being called dispensers, too.

Before audiologists moved into the market, hearing aids were sold by members of the commercial establishment who usually had no qualms about being called dealers. They generally had a high-school education, and were not required to have additional training. Many learned their trade through apprenticeship to an older, more experienced dealer. Until recently, there was no legal licensure or registration for dealers.

However, some form of licensure has been instituted in almost all states now. In some states, a licensed audiologist does not have to get an additional license in hearing aid dispensing. Licensure means that the dispenser has passed a written and practical examination. Feel free to ask to see a license if one is not hanging on the wall.

For the sake of convenience, we will start using the word *dispenser/dealer* when talking about those who used to be just plain dealers; the phrase *dispensing audiologist* will refer to an audiologist who sells hearing aids; the term dispenser will be used when it doesn't make any difference.

Playing this word game won't help you make a decision on which type of dispenser to choose, however, so let's get on with the matter at hand. To whom should you go for a hearing aid? Well, if you have an audiologist's recommendation for a hearing aid, and know of a well-recommended dispenser/dealer in the area, you may get excellent service there. However, if you don't know a dispenser/dealer by reputation, you may be better off buying from a dispensing audiologist. Here's why:

• An audiologist has been licensed by the state, accredited by a national professional group, or both.
• An audiologist will be able to do additional advanced testing of the hearing loss, if necessary.
• Most dispensing audiologists will be able to handle any therapy and training you will need.
• A dispensing audiologist probably won't charge any more than a dispenser/ dealer.

Again, this does not mean that a dispenser/dealer won't do a good job. There are many skilled, competent, and concerned dispenser/dealers in the marketplace. However, you have no guarantee that the dispenser you pick out of the yellow pages will be knowledgeable and conscientious.

On a related note: Physicians have been known, on occasion, to refer a patient directly to a dispenser/ dealer without a complete hearing evaluation. This is generally not a good practice. For one thing, a dispenser who is not an audiologist generally has no training in the complexities of hearing testing, and may not be able to spot or deal with special problems. The evaluation equipment used may not be as sophisticated as an audiologist's.

Each professional, whether an audiologist or not, has his or her own techniques and protocols for fitting hearing aids. So the descriptions given here may not be exactly what you experience. That doesn't make your experience wrong. There are just several philosophies out there. The process for getting aids will also vary depending on the type you are getting, i.e., standard analog, analog hybrid programmable, or 100% digital. So first here are a few things that may be done for all. Then the variations will be discussed.

- The dispenser will be sure you have a recent (within 4-6 months) hearing evaluation and medical clearance or a waiver (as mentioned elsewhere the requirement for medical clearance may change soon). You may also be asked what, if any, your financial restrictions are. Don't be afraid to let them know if you are on a limited budget. They need to know that in planning which fitting is best for you. You also need to be honest about cosmetics, if asked. Hearing aid decisions should not be made based on vanity, and you shouldn't make up your mind ahead of time what the aids should look like, but if you know that you will *never* wear a BTE style, for example, let them know in the beginning.

• The dispenser will interview you about your communication problems and your thoughts and attitudes about hearing aids. You may even be given a standardized questionnaire concerning current problems and expectations, which will be used later to determine if the aids gave improvement and satisfaction.

• The dispenser will ask you to make judgments on what is the most comfortable level of loudness of speech and of tones, and also the level at which the loudness becomes uncomfortable. There are no right and wrong answers here. It is just what sounds good or bad to you. Is it too soft, too loud, or just right?

• The dispenser may have something called a video-otoscope, which is like a live video of the inside of your ear canal. It is not necessary to a good fitting, but it is entertaining to the client to see the inside of their own ears. It helps in counseling you about your problem and is excellent advertising for the office. In some cases where there are unique factors in your anatomy, especially with CIC aids, this can be useful for the fitting. Also, some audiologists are now trained to remove small amounts of non-impacted earwax. This instrument can be a big help in the process.

• Many offices now have an instrument to do real ear measurements where a tiny microphone is inserted inside the ear canal (painless procedure) near the eardrum and the unique acoustic characteristics of each person's ear are determined by putting sounds from a loudspeaker into the ear.

The client does nothing except sit still. The measurements are used when determining the optimal characteristics of the hearing aids. With most aids, the measurements can be taken again with the hearing aid in place to verify that the aid is producing the appropriate sound at the eardrum.

• Some offices use a "master hearing aid" where temporary earmolds are put in your ears so the dispenser can try various levels of sound and different pitch responses while you make subjective evaluations as to what is more clear and natural. It is rather like a visit to the optometrist who dials lenses in front of you so you can tell which allows you to see the best. You can also experience first hand, the advantage of two aids over one.

• Using all the above information, the dispenser will discuss recommendations with you concerning one vs. two hearing aids, the style of hearing aids, and the technology. You will have to be directly involved in decisions which are not dictated by your ears or your hearing loss. The dispenser will tell you what is required, but will leave options up to you after supplying you with the information.

• You will have impressions taken for making your personalized earmolds for BTE aids, or the shell of the aid itself for ITE, ITC, or CIC aids. A putty-like material will be put in your ear with a syringe or something like a caulking gun. It will be left in your ear for about 5-7 minutes until it hardens and is then removed. However, this is not a foolproof process and the mold may not fit perfectly the first time, especially with CIC aids. Since most impressions are sent away and take about a week to come back, additional impressions can prolong the fitting process.

If you are getting standard analog aids, regardless of style, the results of all the measurements and tests will be used, often with a mathematical formula or fitting chart, to determine the optimal characteristics of your hearing aids. You will return to the office in 1-2 weeks for the actual fitting of the aids. Once they are in your ears and checked for inappropriate feedback, their performance will be verified. This also helps to determine what adjustments need to be made. The dispenser may do any or all of these things:

- ask you about comfort of the aids—do they pinch or rub? Do they feel secure in your ear?
- find your most comfortable and uncomfortable loudness levels with the hearing aid in place
- do real ear measurements with the aid in place
- take another audiogram (tell me when you hear the tones even if they are very soft) in front of a loudspeaker with the aid in place
- ask you to repeat word lists with the aid in place
- any of the above with both aids in place

Following these checks, you should have an orientation to learn about the aids. The dispenser should work with you until you understand how to put them on and take them off, check the battery, operate the controls, and care for the instruments. The orientation should also include hints on how to get used to the aids (such as the suggestions outlined in Chapter 6), and a recommended schedule for breaking them in. You will also at this time be given a user *instructional brochure*, which explains all these things in words and pictures. The brochure will carry a warning about irritation from the earmold: some minor irritation is possible at first, but if soreness or irritation persists the earmold must be adjusted. Also, as the brochure will explain, some people are allergic to the substance in the earmold (see chapter 6). If that's the case, you will need to buy a special kind of mold. You will also be notified that you may experience quite a bit of wax accumulation, also explained in Chapter 6. There is one more warning in this brochure: if the output of the aid exceeds a certain level, it could cause additional hearing loss. Don't let this worry you unduly, because very few hearing aids extend to this extreme maximum output, and if you do need this type of power, the audiologist will have already discussed it with you.

You should ask any questions you have. Be sure to take advantage of your time with the dispenser, because you are paying for this service in the cost of the aids. Whatever you do, don't pretend to understand when you really don't. If you're having difficulty with the aids in the dispenser's office, things will only get worse once you're home.

You will probably return in the near future (within three weeks, usually) to have your progress and the hearing aids checked by the dispenser. In the meantime, you should call on the telephone or make another visit if you experience difficulty. Do not hesitate to take these opportunities if you need help; it is part of what you paid for. Be sure to return for this visit. Forty percent of hearing aids require some sort of modification or adjustment by the dispenser or the manufacturer to get the best results.

If you are getting the more high tech hybrid programmable or 100% digital aids, there is much more counseling and interviewing about your lifestyle and the need for various technologies. The three tiers or generations of analog, hybrid programmable and digital programmable aids are described in detail. Decisions must be made on such things as: automatic vs. manual volume control, remote control vs. buttons on the aid itself, use of directional/dual microphones, style of aid, etc.

Following your participation in all this, the aids are usually ordered with a return appointment in 1-2 weeks. Some offices use temporary earmolds and BTE aids to give you an idea of what the actual aided sound is like, knowing that if you order an ITE, ITC, or CIC aid, it will be slightly different. You shouldn't be nervous about ordering aids without trying them on because the computer programming makes the aids you actually get very flexible during the fitting process.

On your return visit, the aids will be fitted and checked for comfort. Most are very small and should be so comfortable after awhile that you have to put your hand up to your ear to be sure they are there. The digital aids will be wired to a computer while you are wearing them. What happens then will depend on the computer program for that particular brand of aid. But basically there will be a series of voices, tones, noises, and/or speech in noise. You will be asked to make subjective judgments about loudness (both comfortable and uncomfortable) and quality.

Some dispensers will ask you to repeat words, or indicate when you hear soft sounds in front of a loudspeaker. It is unlikely that you will have the real ear measurements with this type of aid on. Sometimes they will check the aid for feedback by getting louder at each pitch band. Be sure to ask to try out the aids with the telephone in the dispenser's office. The telephone circuit may need to be adjusted also.

Once the adjustments are made, the dispenser will spend time teaching you care and maintenance of the aids, describing a plan for getting used to the aids, and discussing warranties and payment plans. There is a lot more participation on your part with high tech aids, but it is not difficult to do.

Return visits for all types of aids are a must. A few good dispensers actually call you in 1-2 days to find out how you are doing, but most see you in about a week to follow your progress, listen to success stories (hopefully) and make adjustments for any problems. Remember though, it can't be fixed if the dispenser doesn't know there is a problem. And they need to know specifics like when, where, with whom, how often, and exactly what was wrong. So write down comments during the week to take with you on your next visit.

The big advantage of high tech aids is that they can be re-programmed for initial adjustments, for changes in hearing loss, and for changes in lifestyle. (You may even want to look a few years down the road, at the possibility of moving into a retirement center where most activities occur in groups, a very difficult listening environment. This is where high tech aids will pay off.) The visits for re-programming should be free for at least six months and preferably a year. After that there will be a charge.

Regardless of the style or type, your hearing aids will be sold to you on a thirty-day trial basis, or with a thirty to forty-five day money back guarantee. On the trial basis, you pay a minimal fee until after the thirty-day period; if you're not satisfied you may elect to return the aids. The thirty-day money back guarantee is much more common and follows much the same procedure, except you put up the money first. Most dispensers operate on one of these two plans, and it is worth your while to do business with one who does. Be aware that if you return the aids, the dispenser will keep about 6-15% of the cost as a cancellation fee, which is reasonable since the dispenser has put in a great deal of time and will have some return costs as well.

Now comes the big question: How much will a hearing aid cost? It varies from $500 for a very basic no frills single aid to $6,000 for two high tech digital aids. At the turn of the century, following were average costs of aids by style and type of aid:

Non-programmable analog:
- BTE & ITE @ $800
- ITC @ $950
- CIC @ $1,400

Programmable:
- BTE & ITE @ $1,300-1,600
- ITC @ $1,450-1,850
- CIC @ $1,850-2,100

Totally digital:
- BTE & ITE @ $2,300
- ITC @ $2,400
- CIC @ $2,700

Another factor concerns the services offered, which are included in the total cost. When you sit down to discuss financial matters with the dispenser, it is vital that you determine what services are included. If some essential services are not part of the total price, you may not be getting the bargain you expected when you were quoted the low price. The total price should include:

- the cost of the hearing aid(s) itself
- the cost of the earmold(s)
- one pack of batteries
- any adjustments to the aid or mold
- counseling and orientation
- return visits until you are satisfied—at least one or two
- the warranty on the aid(s), usually for one year

These are the basic services that should be included; others may also be provided. If some extra services come with the package, you might take them into account when comparison shopping.

True, these services do drive up the cost of a hearing aid. Remember though, that for anyone in business, time is money—and quite a bit of the dispenser's time will be spent on your testing, orientation, and return visits.

This is not to say that you shouldn't expect a good buy, especially now that you're aware of the services that should be included with the purchase price. You may wish to keep this book with you when you talk with dispensers; if they provide all the services listed, you can now compare on the basis of price alone and judge the best bargain.

If you visit or telephone several dispensers, you will note from signs in the window or ads in the yellow pages that they often specialize in one, two, or three brands. When dispensers do a great amount of business with one manufacturer, they can generally get a better wholesale price. They will also be more familiar with the individual aid, and may be able to handle minor repairs themselves, without having to send the aid to the factory for service.

In any event, you will probably get the most for your money if you stick to major brands; a list of them follows. If an audiologist recommends a brand that is not on this list, it does not mean there's something wrong with the brand, or that someone's trying to pull a fast one on you. The hearing aid industry is changing rapidly, and what may be a minor brand when this list was compiled, could corner the market in a few years. Just because a firm isn't a major seller, it doesn't indicate that its product is shoddy; it does mean that professionals in the field have had less experience with the product and won't place as much confidence in it as a well-known name brand.

Major Hearing Aid Manufacturers
(in alphabetical order)

Argosy	Electone
Audiotone	General Hearing
Beltone	Instruments
Bernafon-Maico	GN ReSound

Lori-Unitron
Magnatone
Micro-Tech
Miracle Ear
NuEar
Omni
Oticon
Otosonic
Philips
Phonak
Qualitone
Rexton
Rion
Siemens
Sonic Innovations
Starkey
Telex
United Hearing Systems
Widex

Finally, there is one important point that must be stressed: *If you buy two hearing aids, you should not pay double the price.* Never! Remember that the price you pay includes a hefty markup for the dispenser's time. The amount of time spent in giving you an orientation and teaching you to use the aid does not suddenly double when you wear two of them. You should get *at least* $50 off the second aid.

Unfortunately, dispensers have been known to get away with simply doubling the price on a customer who buys two aids. To make sure you're getting a fair price, when you buy one aid or two, it's a good idea to ask the dispenser to "unbundle" the price—that is, to give you a breakdown of what each piece of the package is costing you. That way, you know exactly what you're paying for. Dispensers are certainly entitled to a fair profit; they couldn't stay in business otherwise—but by the same token, you have a right to get your money's worth when you make such a substantial investment.

After you have purchased a hearing aid, you may want to buy one or more handy devices that make coping with your hearing loss a bit easier; some of those devices will be featured in the next chapter. First, here are some questions frequently asked about buying hearing aids:

How do I check the qualifications of the dispenser/dealer?
The dispenser's license should be posted in the office. It may be a license in audiology, a license in hearing aid dispensing, or both. Look for some current certificates of continuing education as well. Many hearing aid dealers are "board certified", a credential which is granted, following an exam given by the International Hearing Society, a trade association. But this is not a legal credential. Of course a call to the local better business bureau can't hurt.

I'm going to buy a new aid soon. Will the dispenser give me a trade-in on my old aid?
Very rarely. The aid won't do the dispenser any good, other than being used as a loaner after it is reconditioned (if it is a BTE). In most states, it can't be sold. You would be wise to keep the old aid as a spare if it is still working. It may not be a good fit anymore, but it is better than nothing if your new aids need repair. There are organizations which collect used BTE aids and turn in the other styles to a company for spare parts. Check with your dispenser. Whatever you do, don't give the aid to a friend who has a hearing problem. Although they are not as specific as eyeglasses, hearing aids are prescribed to fit particular hearing problems. An inappropriate aid is worse than useless: it can cause so much frustration that your friend may throw it away and decide never to try a hearing aid again.

Are all the warranties on hearing aids for only one year?
A few companies now have standard warranties for two, three, or even four years; however, most are still for one year. For an additional charge, some companies will extend the warranty on aids. Extended warranties are usually a good idea since

hearing aid repairs, unless a minor problem, are almost always at least $100. ITE and ITC aids often need re–casing as your ear canal stretches. That can cost almost $100 as well, and is covered in warranties. You can also get insurance from an independent insurance carrier for such things as loss, theft, or accidental damage. The cost will depend on the style of the aid, age of the aid, and the level of technology. This is often not a bad idea because the warranty may not cover those circumstances, but first check:

• exactly what your warranty does cover
• how long and at what cost the warranty can be extended
• your home owner's policy to see if it covers your aids

Are hearing aids dated?

Yes, but your dispenser may have to show you the code. An aid that is dated in the current year is best, but one dated in the previous year is usually okay to purchase if you are buying within the first few months of the next year.

{ 10 }
Other Helpful Devices

As we mentioned before, a hearing aid is just what the name implies—an aid. It does not restore normal hearing, and there are some situations in which it may be of limited help, especially if you don't get high tech aids. (For example, several people all talking at once; a lot of background noise; a sermon, play, or concert; talking on the telephone.) There are also times when you aren't wearing your hearing aid(s) but you still need to hear, such as when you're in bed or in the shower, and the telephone, doorbell, or smoke alarm rings, or an intruder tries to get in. Or, you may have a loss so severe that even a hearing aid does not help you hear the sounds you want or need to hear.

This chapter is about devices beyond hearing aids that can be very helpful in the above situations. These devices can mean the difference between just getting along and a much easier and finer quality of life. They are relatively inexpensive considering the convenience and enjoyment they will afford. You deserve them.

The Americans with Disabilities Act (ADA), which was enacted about a decade ago, makes it mandatory for most work places and public places to be accessible to the disabled, including those with communication disabilities. Thus, the use of the electronic devices (auxiliary aids) described in this chapter is not just appropriate in your home. It is appropriate in offices, hospitals, hotels, theaters, airports, etc. Even courtrooms are affected where the court reporter system can be utilized.

The idea behind the ADA is to prohibit discrimination against people with disabilities in four areas:

1. Employment settings where otherwise qualified persons must have reasonable conditions in applying, hiring, firing, training, advancement.

2. State and local government agencies and public services, where individuals with disabilities cannot be excluded from participation in programs or activities. All government owned places must have visual alarms, assistive devices, amplified phones and TTY's in phone banks.

3. This includes public transportation on buses and trains; public institutions such as restaurants; stores, stadiums, libraries, hotels/motels, museums, theaters, parks, day care centers, private schools, doctors' offices and private transportation services. They must minimize any direct threat to health and safety and make reasonable accommodation or install auxiliary aids.

4. Telecommunications that provide round the clock relay services as described later in this chapter.

There has been a recent Supreme Court decision that said the ADA is not applicable if the disability can be corrected. So, if you are challenged because you have hearing aids, be sure to tell them that the aids don't help in many situations. Thus, you are still entitled to helpful devices. You may have to refer them to your audiologist if you are still denied access.

One benefit of the American free enterprise system is the fact that there will never be a shortage of gadgets to buy. For those with hearing loss, there are a wide variety of gizmos that flash, vibrate, print, and amplify. Use of them can make life a bit easier even if you might be able to get along without them. A good example of a device to make life a little easier and more enjoyable is *closed-captioned television.*

Television Assistive Devices

Even if you hear well enough to understand most of what's being said on your favorite shows, listening to the audio is still likely to be a strain. And trying to follow a TV show will be almost impossible if you hear very poorly. Foreign accents, background music, or lots of action where you can't see faces will make things worse. Closed captioning relieves this strain by printing out subtitles—the general idea of what's being said—as shown in Figure 10.1. It takes a while to be comfortable with reading the captions, so don't give up prematurely.

All the major television networks, as well as some independent stations, cable TV systems, and Canadian broadcasters, have been using a format called Line 21, to program closed-captioned television; you can find out which programs are captioned from most television program listings, including TV Guide, which uses a special symbol to indicate closed-captioned programs. There are many children's shows now being captioned. Live shows, speeches, and sports events are captioned in "real time"—the speech is immediately typed into a machine like a court stenographer uses and it appears on the screen one or two seconds delayed. A text channel gives a summary of news, sports, cultural, political, and medical information as well as schedules of upcoming programs.

All new televisions with a 13" or bigger screen are now made with the caption system built in. You just have to turn the captioning on if you want it. If you have an older television, you can buy an adaptor that can be turned on and off so the television can be seen without captions, but an adaptor can cost $200, so why not get a new TV?

The captions are about a half-inch high when they're on a nineteen-inch television screen. To insure legibility, the area immediately behind the captions is blacked out.

There are also home videocassette movies that are closed captioned, such as those produced by RCA/Columbia Home Entertainment, and you can tape the captions directly onto your home VCR.

The National Association For The Deaf provides a free captioned film loaner program through which films are sent directly to your home. Contact them at: Captioned Films/Video Program, National Association For The Deaf, 1447 E Main Street, Spartenburg, South Carolina 29307; voice 800-237-6213, TTY 800-237-6819, fax 800-538-5636; www.cfv.org. A website on which to buy captioned videos is in the appendix concerning the Internet.

In the future, look for a possible new development in captioning. Virtual vision sport glasses, originally designed as a personal TV worn on the face, are being modified to display closed captioning on eyeglasses wherever it is offered. And in movie houses, plans are being made for closed captions to be seen on small panels attached to the seats.

Remember, closed captioning units, like hearing aids and many of the other devices useful to the hearing impaired, are tax deductible.

There are some other devices available to those who have trouble understanding the dialog on TV programs (a very common problem even among people who have only mild losses; remember that the sound coming from a television speaker is distorted to begin with, and not accompanied by as many visual cues as in real life). One such device sends the audio signal direct-

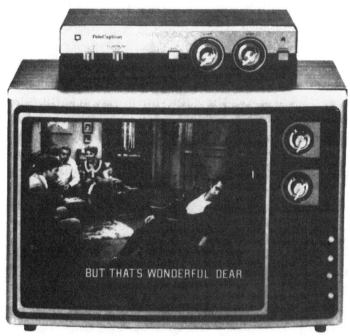

Figure 10.1. Closed captioned television. Closed caption television allows viewers to read most dialogue of most programs. The adaptor seen on the top of the television in this photo is no longer necessary for televisions made after 1998. (Photo courtesy of National Captioning Institute, Inc.)

ly into an earpiece worn by the *hearing impaired* person. Unlike the standard earphone on a television, some of these instruments don't cut out the speaker, so others can watch television with you. The volume control for your earpiece can be adjusted separately from the TV volume control. Prices for this unit—and most of the equipment described in this chapter—vary widely, so it's a good idea to call several hearing aid dispensers (who would most likely order this type of gear from a manufacturer).

Another device for the television is a microphone hooked to an infra–red light emitter. A receiver worn by the listener picks up the light, which actually carries a sound signal from the television. The signal is amplified and played back through the headphones. Now, you can hear the television well while the volume is turned to a level comfortable for others in the room. The system has excellent fidelity and is easy to install. Also, remember that while you are listening under those headphones, the noise in the room around you is blocked out and won't interfere as much. An infra-red emitter and receiver can be found for as low as $100, but a quality system is $200–$300. You can get an adapter to put the signal through your own hearing aid via a telecoil (see below) and an inductance neckloop.

Assistive Devices for Public Places

Many public places such as churches, theaters, and public meeting rooms have installed infra-red systems for their hearing impaired patrons. The speaker's voice or music is transmitted via infra-red light to special receivers provided by the facility. The impaired person wears the receiver and turns the volume up to a comfortable level. The resulting sound is extremely clear and free of most background noise. There is a problem with interference from sunlight, so use of these systems is limited. Ask at the ticket window how to borrow and to use the units, which should be well advertised. There is no charge, but they may ask to hold a credit card or driver's license for security.

Another slightly more elaborate system that is commonly used in theaters, churches, and classrooms for better reception of voice is a radio-frequency FM system (Figures 10.2 and 10.3). The speaker wears a lavaliere (necklace) or lapel microphone, which is also a tiny radio transmitter. The voice is carried over the air within a 50-to-100 foot radius and is picked up by a receiver about the size of a cigarette package worn by the impaired listener. The voice is amplified and put directly into the person's ear through an earphone or is routed by a wire through their hearing aid. The advantage is a clear, amplified sound with little background noise interference. Many public places have this system installed and will loan out the receivers much like the infra-red devices above. However, many people buy their own to use in other circumstances such as in the car, out to dinner, at a professional office, or with their television. The cost for this system for one person (mike, receiver, and re-charger) is about $250 to $600 depending on the sophistication you need. This system can be invaluable to someone who must frequently listen in situations where a speaker is addressing a large group. It is transportable from place to place and easy to use. If used in a meeting, several microphones can be used or one microphone can be put near the center of a table. Some can even be plugged into a tape recorder for a clear, lasting record of what was said.

You can get an adapter to feed the FM signal into your regular aid, or wear a neckloop of wire that converts the FM signal into electromagnetic waves that are picked up by your T-switch (see below). Microlink is a miniaturized wireless FM receiver and transmitter tht is compatible with many brands of BTE aids. This small cube attaches to the base of the aid and inputs the FM signal.

Personal FM systems are now available that have the receiver devices entirely contained in a behind-the-ear aid so it can be used as a regular hearing aid or as an FM device. While they are expensive—about $1,200—they can be extremely useful and do not have cords or boxes for the listener to wear (but the speaker must still wear a microphone and the listening device has a small antennae).

Other helpful devices for someone with a hearing loss use electromagnetic waves that can be picked up by a T-switch (called T because telephones emit the waves). Many hearing aids are equipped with a T-switch for listening to the telephone. In fact we strongly suggest you ask for a T-switch in the BTE and ITE styles. The extra $50-100 is well worth it. The smaller styles probably don't have enough room for one.

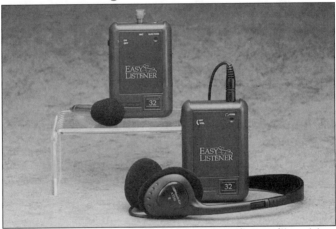

Figure 10.2 A personal FM listening system (transmitter at top, receiver at bottom) can be used with a hearing aid with direct audio input, or with walkman-type earphones, as shown here. (Photo courtesy of Phonic Ear)

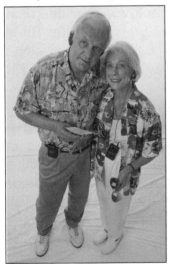

Figure 10.3 The personal FM listening system with transmitter and earphone receiver. (Photo courtesy of Phonic Ear)

Even though the T-switch might not be the answer to all your telephone problems (we'll discuss some alternatives in a moment) it can be very helpful in combination with a system called a loop. How does a loop system work? A microphone picks up, let's say, a sermon. It then feeds the sermon through a powerful system of wires encircling the room. By switching the hearing aid to the T-position while sitting within the wires, you receive a direct feed of an electromagnetic signal. The reception should be better than what you get from the microphone of your aids and will have less background noise. The loop system idea can be applied to a radio or television set, and will feed the audio into a mini loop (about $200) around the person, and thus to the hearing aid via the T-switch. If your aid does not have a T-switch, you can get a pocket-sized inductance receiver with an earphone.

Many churches, lecture rooms, theaters, and concert halls have installed these loop systems. Most of these locations advertise this service; just ask in which section of the room you should sit because the whole room may not be wired. If you don't have a hearing aid with a T-switch, most places will have a receiver you can borrow, and you will be given instructions on how to use it.

Telephone Assistive Devices

The T-switch on hearing aids is very helpful when listening to the telephone. When the switch is in the T position, the aid is no longer sensitive to sound waves. Instead, it amplifies electromagnetic waves produced in the receiver of the telephone. The theory, of course, is that the telephone signal can be transmitted directly into the hearing aid without amplifying any background noise in the room. In practice, though, some older phones do not work well, if at all, with a T-switch. At one time phones were shielded to prevent wiretapping—a good idea, but one that prevented the units from working with a T-switch. If the phone has been manufactured since 1989, it will be T-switch compatible; all corded and cordless phones, according to federal regulation, must accommodate the T-switch.

The quality of a T-switch varies widely from aid to aid. So try yours out at the dispenser's office before you go home with it.

The T-switch is a good idea if you have a compatible

telephone, but it takes awhile to find just the right position of phone and aid. Remember it is the coil inside the hearing aid that is picking up the sound, not your ear, so don't put the phone in it's usual position. Turn the volume up and experiment with putting the phone receiver in different locations near the hearing aid while someone on the other end of the telephone line counts to one hundred. If your loss is very severe, you may need an extra powerful T-switch with a booster. Talk to your dispenser. Telecoils and their various uses have increased overall satisfaction with hearing aids.

To be frank, hearing impaired people and telephones just don't get along well. Use of the telephone is one of the most irksome problems faced by the hearing impaired, for a number of reasons. The biggest problem usually rests in the fact that the normal telephone just isn't loud enough. A device to overcome this dilemma is an amplified telephone equipped with a volume wheel or switch. The wheel or switch, usually located in the center of the hand-held portion of the phone, works just like the volume control on a radio. The advantage of having a volume wheel is that you can turn the phone up as loud as you like, while getting a relatively undistorted signal. Some telephones come with a standard volume increase switch. These are usually not loud enough. Find one made especially for those with hearing loss.

You will, however, usually want to take your hearing aid off when talking into an amplified phone (unless you can use an unaided ear). The only time it's feasible to use a hearing aid without a T-switch to amplify the sound of the telephone is with an ITE, ITC, or CIC aid. These may, however, result in feedback when you hold the receiver up to your ear. Try angling the telephone out a little, or getting a foam or hard plastic ring made for this problem.

There is a charge for the telephone company to

install a volume-wheel-controlled phone (usually about
$25), and a minimal per month rental fee. We suggest
you purchase an amplifier receiver for $35 and install it
yourself, which is fairly easy. Be sure it is compatible
with your telephone—take your phone with you or have
all the information about your phone available when
your purchase the amplifier. Also, remember that if you
depend on an amplified telephone handset, you are
restricted to your own phone; however, when you see a
pay phone marked for handicapped users it will generally be equipped with a volume wheel.

For about $20–30 you can purchase a small coupler
that fits over the listening end of most telephone
receivers and makes the sound louder. It is easily moved
from one phone to another. However, the quality is not
quite as good as a built-in amplifier, and if you forget to
turn the coupler off when you hang up, the batteries
wear out quickly. The couplers are often available in
electronic shops. Be careful of these couplers. Some
don't help and can even hinder your hearing. Try them
out and return if they don't help you. AT&T makes a
good quality portable amplifying unit that you can
request through the phone company. Amplified phone
handsets add about thirty decibels of power—enough
for moderate to severe losses; portable units boost
sound by about twenty-two decibels—enough for mild
to moderate losses. For extra power, use an amplifier
plus the T-switch on your hearing aid.

A good alternative is a whole new telephone. There
are some available which have a choice of different
tones and/or loudness of the ring. The voice level and
pitch can be adjusted to your hearing loss. The numbers
are big and easy to see and push. Some have a visual
ring flasher, as well as the convenience of regular high
tech telephones with memory and redial. One is even
cordless ($100-200).

The advancement of technology in the field of telephones has been a problem for those using hearing aids. In the 1950's when wire-tapping was a problem, the telephone companies installed shields that made telecoils (T-switches) on hearing aids useless. It took many decades to finally rid ourselves of those shields. Then along came fancy models like "dial in the handset", mobile cordless phones, cellular phones and the digital phones which were all major problems for the hearing aid user.

But through the efforts of advocacy groups, most of the problems can be solved. In fact, many solutions have come from the manufacturers of the telephones. Guess they wanted your business. In any case, whenever you purchase a telephone, be sure to ask about hearing aid compatibility. But don't expect the salesperson to always be informed. Insist on trying it out before buying. Sometimes it may require an accessory, like a neck loop, and sometimes the solution is brand-specific. But remember, the government is making new regulations to help you and telephones get along better.

For those who can't use a telephone at all, there's a device called a TTY (teletypewriter). These phones have also been called TDD (telecommunications device for the deaf) and text telephones (TT) in their history. But most recently, TTY tends to be used most (fig. 10.4).

The basic stripped-down model costs less than $200. You type your message in on a typewriter-type keyboard, and it is typed out on a screen on the receiver's TTY. You can also buy a system that prints out the conversation on paper as well. Previously you were limited to calling parties who also have a TTY, but that includes many airlines, hospitals, schools, fire and police stations, and government offices.

But now there are services whereby an operator will receive the TTY message and re-transmit it orally to a party who has only a conventional telephone. Thanks to federal regulation in 1990 all states are required to have these relay services 24 hours a day, which allow someone with a TTY to communicate with people who use a standard phone and vice versa. A communications assistant (CA) is contacted through a toll free number. To find out the number for your area or for more information on the relay systems, look in your local telephone book under "customers with disabilities/ relay service" or dial 411 (nationwide directory assistance).

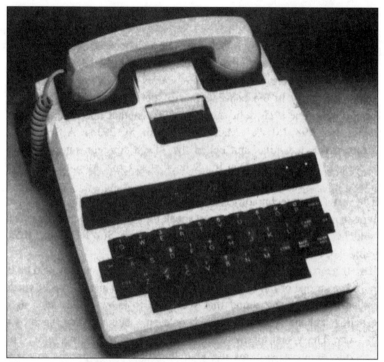

Figure 10.4. A TTY. The message transmitted shows up on the screen above the keyboard. (Photo courtesy of Known Research Inc.)

The CA relays the TTY input to the telephone of the hearing person and then types that person's response. Obviously there are slight delays while the CA types, and there are pre-arranged signals such as saying/typing GA ("go ahead") when you are finished with your part of the message, or saying/typing SK to sign off. The CA will gladly explain the whole process to either party. The CA follows strict confidentiality and there are no records kept of conversations. Local calls are free as is the use of the CA, but long distance calls are billed. TTY customers can apply for special discounts since it takes longer to have a conversation.

Suppose you are hearing impaired enough to need the TTY, but you can speak clearly. Then use a voice over (VO) during the relay call where the CA types the message to you, but you can speak directly rather than typing back. In fact, this system in reverse can also be used for people who hear but can't speak.

A TTY costs between $250 and $600, depending on the conveniences built in. Some units have an answering machine, a printer, or call waiting included in the mechanism.

Household Sound Devices

If your hearing loss is severe enough to require a TTY, you may also be in the market for one or more sound sensor units. These alarms can be made sensitive to almost any sound that you need to know about, such as a doorbell, telephone ring, an intruder, or even a human voice, such as a baby's cry. The visual alarm generally consists of a flashing light. The more complex alarm systems use your home electrical circuits to carry signals so that, without obtrusive wiring, you can have a lamp that flashes in each room ($150-$400). There can be a code of flashes for the different sounds around the house. For example, a telephone ring could be one flash; the doorbell could be three flashes; while the stove timer might be two. Incidentally, unless you are totally deaf the best system for alerting you to an intruder would be a very loud burglar-alarm system. You can even get one that would also ring into your neighbor's house or (in many locations) to the police station, or the central station of the burglar-alarm company.

If you live in a one room apartment, try a knock light: a light that flashes as someone knocks on your door ($50-$75). There is also a strobe light that is integrated into a smoke alarm.

A particular convenience for people who have trouble hearing the phone, is a system that produces a very bright strobe-light flash when the phone rings ($75). You can also purchase a device that vibrates a wristband when the phone is ringing. This device can also alert you to other household sounds.

Vibrators are helpful for people who have trouble waking to an alarm clock. The vibrator usually is connected to the clock and placed under the pillow or mattress; the vibrator replaces the normal alarm buzzer on the clock. You can even have your doorbell hooked into this vibrating system. But before you invest in a sophisticated wake up system, check out some of the old-fashioned wind-up alarm clocks, such as the Baby Ben. These clocks generate quite a bit of noise and will certainly be louder than a buzzer on most electric clocks or clock radios. You may also try a timer that turns on the lights each morning to wake you.

Other Devices
Some others you might want to check into:

• A fax machine—yes, the garden-variety fax is a wonderful tool for the hearing impaired, and you can buy a reasonably good one for $150 or so.

• A (hardwired) personal listening system that operates over a short wire between two people. You can put a microphone on the person speaking and route the output to your ear piece ($100-$150). These are useful for restaurants, car rides, and doctor's offices.

• A telephone answering machine will take a message that can then be amplified and played over and over for better understanding.

• A "blinker buddy" alerts a driver that his turn signal has been left on, as the standard alerting sound in a car is very difficult to hear ($75).

• Siren alert—a device in your vehicle that alerts you to an emergency siren or horn outside.

• A standard intercom system between you and your child's bedroom or playroom or your spouse's work area. Don't depend on hearing from another room even with hearing aids.

Most of the devices are not sold in typical stores, except for ones like a regular burglar alarm or a coupler for your telephone. You can call, write or check the Internet to get free catalogs and order directly from these sources:

ADCO Hearing Products Inc.
5661 S. Curtice Street
Littleton, CO 80120
800-726-0851
fax 303-794-3704
sales@adcohearing.com

General Technologies
7417 Winding Way
Fair Oaks, CA 95628-6701
800-328-6684
fax: 916-961-9823

Harc Mercantile
P.O. box 3055
Kalamazoo, MI 49003-3055
800-445-9968
fax 800-413-5248
www.harcmercantile.com
home@hacofamerica.com

Hear More, Inc.
42 Executive Blvd.
Farmingdale, NY 11735
800-881-4327
fax: 516-752-0689
www.maxiaids.com
sales@hearmore.com

HITEC Group Intl Inc.
8160 Madison Ave.
Burr Ridge, IL 60521
800-288-8303
fax: 630-654-9219
www.hitec.com
dannee@hitec.com

NFSS Communications
8120 Fenton Street
Silver Spring, MD 20910
888-589-6670
fax: 301-589-5153
www.nfss.com
sales@nfss.com

Ultratec Inc.
450 Science Drive
Madison, WI 53711
800-482-2424
fax: 608-238-3008
www.ultratec.com

Williams Sound Corp.
10399 W. 70th Street
Eden Prairie, MN 55344-3459
800-328-6190
fax: 612-943-2174
info@williamssound.com
www.williamssound.com

One final note: When you make plans to purchase any type of device, such as a hearing aid or any instrument described in this chapter, always keep firmly in mind that no gadget will be the cure-all for a hearing impairment. It may make your life easier, but it won't solve all the communication problems that result from a hearing loss. If you don't expect it to, you won't be disappointed.

There are many aspects of communication that won't ever be the same, regardless of what you buy or how much money you spend. Conversation in a noisy restaurant will never be particularly easy, and it probably will always be a bit difficult to hear a distant speaker. But this doesn't mean there's nothing you can do to improve matters—far from it. By practicing a program for better communication, outlined in the next chapter, you can polish your communication skills and effectively cope with all types of everyday situations.

First, let's examine some typical questions about the topic covered in this chapter:

I read somewhere about "hearing ear dogs." Was it a joke?

Not at all. Several firms are training hearing ear dogs (also called signal dogs), usually for people who are totally deaf or have a very severe hearing loss, and live alone. The hearing ear dog is trained to be sensitive to certain noises (such as a doorbell ringing or a baby crying) and to run back and forth between the source of the noise and the dog's master. There are laws in each state concerning the use of these dogs. It costs $3,000 to train one, but they are available to those with hearing loss at $500 or less. There are a few centers around the U.S. that train these dogs. Check with your state association for the deaf or on the Internet at www.assistance-dogs-intl.org

I have trouble hearing the telephone when I'm in another part of the house. What should I do?

The telephone company can install extra ringing devices in other parts of the house; or, of course, you can have another phone installed. Before you call the phone company, though, be sure that the ringing device on your present phone is turned up full blast. The adjustment is underneath the telephone, or on the side of a wall model.

The telephone company also can install a louder ringing device in your phone, or you can even get a ring at a lower pitch, which is easier for you to hear. If your loss is really bad, you may need a system where a light flashes when a telephone rings.

My husband gets angry when he talks to me from downstairs and I don't hear. Will a hearing aid help?

Probably not entirely. Speech from another room is not only soft, but it is distorted. Hearing aids do not allow you to hear very soft sounds. And the distortion won't allow you to understand: Why not install an intercom system in the house so you can always be in touch?

How can I be alerted to a natural or community disaster?

The Federal Communication Commission (FCC) has an Emergency Alert system that requires all television stations to transmit emergency messages in both audio and text modes that do not interfere with other text on the screen.

{ 11 }
Tinnitus

A closely related problem to hearing loss is tinnitus (pronounced either TIN-ih-tus or ti-NIH-tus), which is usually described as ringing or roaring in the ears or head. Some people describe it as the whistling of the wind or a tea kettle, some as a bell or a high pitched tone, others as crickets or locusts, or maybe a seashell held up to the ear. A few have several of these sounds all at once.

Up to 40 million Americans (one in five of the entire population) experience this as a chronic problem at some time in their lives. Most people occasionally experience a sudden dull feeling in the ear, followed by a ringing sound that gradually goes away after 30-60 seconds. That's normal. Some have also experienced ringing in the ears and muffled speech sounds after exposure to really loud sounds like a jet engine, a rock concert, or a gun blast. That's damage to your hearing taking place, but most of it returns and the ringing stops after a few hours.

However, if the noise was very, very loud, or if you continue to be exposed to it again and again, the hearing loss and tinnitus may get worse and become permanent. (A recent threat in this area is automotive air bags, which can have up to a 175 dB sound when they deploy.)

Twenty percent of those 40 million people with tinnitus suffer from long term tinnitus which can last for hours, days, weeks, or a lifetime. They are concerned enough to consult a healthcare professional. About one to two million in this group find the disorder so debilitating, painful or at least severely annoying, that they cannot function well on a day-to-day basis.

For these people the tinnitus may be constant or intermittent. It can be subjectively loud or soft. It can be in one ear, both ears, or just "somewhere in the head." It may be with them all the time, or just noticed in quiet places like a bedroom or a hearing testing booth. It can be worse under certain conditions such as psychological stress, or following a loud activity like mowing the lawn.

Some people learn to ignore the tinnitus once they realize it is not a danger signal. It becomes part of normal body noises like swallowing, digestion, and breathing. It becomes a handicap when it is severe enough to interfere with psycho-social functioning, i.e., daily activities. People who experience tinnitus have problems with sleep, concentration, understanding speech, persistence on a task, annoyance/irritation, despair/depression, headaches, stress and even drug dependence from some of the treatments.

What is tinnitus? Where does it come from? The simple answer is, we don't know for sure. We know it is a symptom, but we are usually not sure of what. There are lots of theories, but none proven. There are a lot of treatments, but none consistently successful. In fact, the reason why tinnitus is so tough to conquer is because there is no proven mechanism causing it; there are no objective measures of it; it is not a disease but a symptom; it involves the central nervous system as well as the ear; and it is impacted by the emotional system. Much like pain, tinnitus is subjective, invisible, and affected by extraneous events.

Rarely, people have what is called *objective tinnitus,*

which is when the physician can actually hear it also. That is typically a vascular problem or muscle spasm and can usually be fixed.

We do know that tinnitus often accompanies hearing loss due to noise exposure, toxic drugs, metabolic imbalances, tumors, or aging. About 10% of tinnitus sufferers have normal hearing as determined by standard hearing testing but, in fact, if hearing were tested into the very high pitches, probably most people with tinnitus would find they had some abnormal hearing.

Sometimes the tinnitus is a symptom of ear disease, or even general ailments like cardiovascular disease or underactive thyroid gland; these problems, of course, should receive medical attention. Some people report the onset of tinnitus at menopause, with *TMJ* (jaw misalignment) problems, following manipulation by a chiropractor, or after head or neck trauma. Tinnitus can be induced by or exacerbated by large amounts of aspirin, analgesics, quinine, diuretics, caffeine, alcohol, nicotine or sodium. Also, the cause could be something as simple as impacted ear wax. So be sure to make your physician the first step you take in dealing with frequent tinnitus.

One current theory about the origin of tinnitus is similar to the phantom limb syndrome—where someone who has lost an arm or a leg still feels sensations such as pain or burning from where the limb was. The theory suggests that a hearing loss from a problem in the ear causes less transmission of information to the brain. This causes the brain to "turn up the power" in an effort to get more input, so we hear more body noises. Some think that the brain actually produces its own sounds when it is not getting stimulated at certain pitches by the ears. Some high tech medical imaging of the brain supports this theory. Of course this is one kind of tinnitus, and there are others whose origin may be abnormal nerve discharges, deficient metabolic chemicals, etc.

The many possible origins are what makes it tough, if not impossible, to cure.

So, if you have tinnitus, are you doomed to live with it? Well, yes, and no. Don't let a physician or audiologist tell you to "learn to live with it" and send you on your way because there is nothing they can do. Maybe there is no medical or surgical cure, or maybe this professional does not deal with tinnitus, but there is help. Find someone who does deal with it. One way to accomplish this is to contact the American Tinnitus Association, P.O. Box 5, Portland OR, 97207-0005, telephone 1-800-634 8978, e-mail tinnitus@ata.org, or on the Internet at www.ata.org.

So what kind of help is available? There are many varieties of what are called *tinnitus patient management procedures*. (Note that the patient is managed, not the tinnitus.) The process should start with an evaluation by a hearing healthcare professional. An interview helps define the problem by asking how long the tinnitus has been experienced, the behaviors it affects, patients' attitudes and thoughts about it, and foods, activities or situations that affect it. You might also be asked to rate the severity of your tinnitus on scales of 1-10. A tinnitus match might be done where you are asked to match the loudness and pitch of your tinnitus with sounds from earphones. A full hearing evaluation will be done as well.

Interestingly enough, the tinnitus is usually quite soft (only slightly louder than the softest sound the person can hear), despite its annoying effect. The pitch is usually very high (above 3000 Hz), sometimes even way above the pitch range of speech.

The healthcare professional might also perform a procedure where you will listen to a soft noise for awhile and see if it covers up the tinnitus. This is called *masking* and might be important in deciding on a treatment for you. There may even be some relief from the tinnitus for a short time after the noise is taken away. This is called residual inhabition or post-masking recovery.

After this evaluation for tinnitus, be sure that any physical factors for your tinnitus have been eliminated or treated by your physician. For example, about half of those with TMJ (temporal-mandibular joint) problems have tinnitus. Through painless procedures of stimulation of the muscles and joints of the jaw, it is claimed that 50-95% are helped. However, if it has been determined that there are no physical factors causing your tinnitus that should receive medical attention and there is a good idea of the characteristics of your particular tinnitus, there are several treatments/coping mechanisms that can be tried. Some of the more drastic ones like surgery (which rarely works) and prescription medications like Xanax (most of which have side effects) should be saved as last resort.

Probably the best place to start is by educating the sufferer about the nature of tinnitus and giving reassurance that it is probably not a warning of impending deafness, or of impending grave illness, and is not a sign of insanity. There is no evidence that tinnitus will get worse, and it does not have to result in lack of control over your life. This knowledge alone can allow many people to put it in the back of their mind and forget it most of the time.

Also, there are some simple and effective strategies that you can begin to use right now:

  • Avoid very quiet situations where there is no background noise to cover up the tinnitus. Get a clock radio for going to sleep and waking up, or an instrument that plays sounds of nature like wind, waves, and rain. A pillow loudspeaker might be a good idea if you don't sleep alone. A product that costs $50 and can be well worth it to tinnitus sufferers is sound pillow, a wafer thin micro-stereo speaker in a full size pillow with speaker jacks for radios, TV's or stereos. Call toll free 877-846-6488 or www.soundpillow.com.

• Avoid very loud situations, which might make the tinnitus worse. This includes recreational as well as occupational noise.

• Try to avoid psychological stress or try stress management courses because stress makes it worse.

• Examine your diet to determine any exacerbating factors such as high salt, alcohol, or caffeine. Even high cholesterol diets have been studied as culprits. Go off or reduce these items for several weeks and then suddenly start them again.

• Try ginko biloba; some people have reported good results. But check with your doctor because this is a blood thinner and might interact with other medications. Other suggested supplements have been B complex vitamins, zinc, and calcium. But again, be careful as there are no recommended dosages and no research evidence of success.

• While we're thinking of alternative medicine, many people have reported relief from acupuncture, but even acupuncturists admit it only works on a few. Hypnosis and electro-stimulation have also been tried with some success and some failure.

• Some doctors prescribe sleep aid drugs or anti-depressants.

• Relaxation techniques and attention diversion are methods of self-help, or you can consult your audiologist or a counselor to help you.

Tinnitus itself can cause tension and nervousness, and it can become worse during periods of physical or emotional stress or fatigue. In either case, relaxation can help. Try breathing exercises where you take deep breaths with your eyes closed. With the exhalation, try to relax all the muscles. Mentally focus on the breathing activity.

To perform progressive muscular relaxation, sequentially tense and then relax various muscle groups throughout the body. Sit or lie comfortably with your eyes closed. Start with the right, then the left foot, lower legs, upper legs, back, stomach, shoulders, chest, biceps, lower arms, hands, neck, jaw, forehead. Try to become aware of particular areas prone to tension. Do a spot check on these areas and deliberately relax as soon as tension increases. Once you are comfortable relaxing in a quiet secluded place, move to different locations to relax. This can be useful for other tension producing situations such as traffic, waiting in line, or being yelled at.

If you can learn to focus your attention away from your tinnitus and on other things both inside and outside your body, your awareness of the tinnitus will diminish. Try this exercise: close your eyes and focus your attention on your breathing. Note the in and out phase and the length of each, the moment of direction change, etc. Now focus on your feet. Note the sensations in your left and then your right foot, and now in each toe separately. Notice that when you focus on one thing, the other recedes into the background.

Pay attention to your awareness as if it were a flashlight to highlight whatever sensation you wish. Allow your awareness to go back and forth from your breathing to your feet. Now change focus from inside you to outside of you, such as temperature or sensations on the outside of your skin. Notice the sounds in your head. Shift back to the sensations in your feet or your breathing. Notice thoughts and images that come to mind, and see how they interfere with sensations and awareness. See how you can only focus on one thing at a time. Try going back and forth between the internal noises and the external stimulation. When you focus on other things, your attention is diverted from the tinnitus.

One form of this attention diversion is *imagery*, where you imagine a situation or place that is pleasant. This can be a mental visualization of something pleasant that sounds similar to your tinnitus—wind in the trees, waves on the shore, steak sizzling on a barbeque, cicadas in the trees, waterfalls, a stream, a roaring fire in a fireplace, a piece of music. If there is no auditory match, think of a perfect place to escape in difficult times. To visualize an image, you must use all your sensations: sight, sound, smell, touch, taste. When paying attention to a scene in your imagination, other sensations will subside into the background. If you can control your attention focus, the tinnitus should be less distressing. This might be especially helpful with sleep disturbance.

If the techniques above don't provide relief and you have a hearing loss, even one that you hardly notice, try hearing aids! As demonstrated by a quiet room, tinnitus seems worse when there is nothing to cover it up. Try plugging your ears and your tinnitus will likely seem to get louder. Your brain reacts to not receiving information from the ears because of a real or simulated hearing loss, even within a narrow pitch range.

Hearing aids on both ears (if you only put an aid in the ear where you hear the tinnitus, you will probably then hear it in the other ear) actually partially or completely mask out the tinnitus for many people. If it does not work for you, or if you don't have a hearing loss, a masker may be the answer. This device looks like a hearing aid, but produces a soft waterfall-like sound which covers up the tinnitus but does not block other sound from entering the ear. Yes, this is substituting one sound for another, but psychologically it is easier for most people to tolerate a sound over which they have control. DTM by Petroff Audio Technologies (www.tinnitushelp.com, tel. 818-716-6166, fax 818-704-9976), is a personal masking system for temporary relief of tinnitus. It is a series of CD's with a workbook to mask the tinnitus and promote relaxation.

With hearing aids, you also get the additional benefit, and maybe pleasant surprise, of hearing better. Besides, both hearing aids and maskers can have a bonus for many people called residual inhabition where the tinnitus is gone or reduced for hours after the instrument is taken off. About 12% of people get relief with hearing aids alone, 21% with maskers alone, and 67% with a combination unit, according to the Oregon Tinnitus Center. But in a few cases these devices can actually aggravate tinnitus.

There are management procedures which are more psychologically based. One is cognitive-behavior therapy. It involves determining the emotional reactions to tinnitus, identifying thoughts and situations associated with each emotion, and then learning to modify inappropriate thoughts and behaviors. The concept is that the tinnitus is real and may be permanent but reaction to it is the true source of the problem. Therefore it is manageable and can be modified if the significance or threat of tinnitus is removed, and attention can then be directed elsewhere. This therapy changes the way one interprets thoughts and feelings by removing inappropriate beliefs, anxieties, and fears. It helps reduce such behaviors as:

• Focusing on tinnitus and ignoring other input. (Focusing on tinnitus makes it worse, but tinnitus is not noticed when you are focused on something else.)

• Assuming other's thoughts about you. ("They must think I'm crazy.")

• Jumping to conclusions with negative expectations. ("I'll die from lack of sleep if this tinnitus keeps up.")

• Ignoring positive experiences that conflict with negative views. ("When I'm absorbed in a good book, movie or conversation, the tinnitus is gone.")
• Treating negative events as intolerable catastrophes. ("My life is ruined because I can't concentrate on my work.")
• Assuming blame. ("If I hadn't gone to the rock concert, I wouldn't have tinnitus.")

Cognitive restructuring is changing the way one thinks. It is based on the concept that there are three aspects of reactions to events: the situation or event itself; our thoughts/perceptions/expectations of the event; and our emotions/behaviors in reaction to the event. By restructuring or changing the second aspect, we can impact the third. For example:

Event: An Offer of Help in Pumping Gas
          scenario #1
• Thoughts/perceptions: I feel like such an idiot that I can't do this. This person must think I am really stupid.
• Emotional consequences: feelings of negativity, depression, low self esteem.
          vs. scenario #2
• Thoughts/perceptions: isn't it nice that there are helpful people around when I need them!
• Emotional consequences: positive attitude toward being helped, feeling cared about.

Event: Having Tinnitus
          scenario #1
• Thoughts/perceptions: why me? Why do I have to suffer? It's not fair.
• Emotional consequences: feelings of frustration, despair, depression.

vs. scenario #2
- Thoughts/perception: the noise is a nuisance, but there are so many other good things in life to enjoy.
- Emotional consequences: feelings of optimism, healthy acceptance of a problem that can be dealt with.

Event: Being Invited to a Social Function
scenario #1
- Thoughts/perceptions: I can't go. I can't hear. The tinnitus will get worse and I'll just make a fool of myself.
- Emotional consequences: feelings of anxiety and frustration, socially inhibitive tension.

vs. scenario #2.
- Thoughts/perceptions: oh good! When I am out socially there are too many distractions to be bothered by my tinnitus and if it gets worse, it will settle down later.
- Emotional consequences: positive outlook, excitement about an event, self-assured attitude.

Once reactions are identified, examined, and more positive alternatives are found, tinnitus becomes much easier to live with.

The second psychological approach also involves some instrumentation. Tinnitus retraining therapy (TRT), a habituation therapy, was developed in the early 1990's. Therapists should be specially trained for this protocol. The primary goal is to interfere with the person's reaction to and perception of tinnitus. This involves the use of low level noise generators which, unlike maskers, do not cover up the tinnitus, but just get people in the habit of listening to low level sound so there is less reaction to the tinnitus noise.

The concept is that people may or may not choose to attend to their tinnitus just as they may or may not attend to the sound of their refrigerator, the clock tick-ing, or the traffic outside their house. This habituation, in which the person chooses not to react to the sound and not to attend to it, can take a long time. A common response after treatment of 1-2 years is, "I know my tin-nitus is there, but it doesn't bother me anymore. Often I am not even aware of it unless I purposely think of it or I'm under a lot of stress."

The first part of this therapy involves counseling to learn about tinnitus and take away the tension, fear and anxiety, thus the emotional reaction. Counseling is fol-lowed by very soft sound distraction, accomplished by wearing the noise generators 6-16 hours a day. The per-son will eventually ignore the sound just like they do household noise. This hopefully allows the brain to selectively filter out the similar tinnitus noise, at some point removing the perception of the tinnitus from the person's consciousness, at which point the special pro-cedure and noise generator are no longer required.

There are some pretty complex biological/physio-logical explanations that go with this, but the average reader doesn't want to know them. For the curious, con-tact the American Tinnitus Association who can refer you to centers around the country trained in this proce-dure. Some of these centers claim 85% of their patients experience some improvement, but the cost can be about $3,000.

Which road is best for you to follow? As with any health problem, it's tough to be out there on your own. That's why personal contact with a local support group helps. But if there are none in your area, contact the American Tinnitus Association. They can put you in touch with support people either through the telephone or e-mail. They can send you loads of good information, and they can refer you to professionals/clinics who take tinnitus seriously. Look for someone who is articulate and can explain things well enough for you to easily understand. Do they seem to want to know and care about your particular problem? Find someone with previous experience in dealing with tinnitus who appears to be in charge with a clear therapy plan, but lets you participate in the discussions and decisions. Are they realistic about outcome, but have hope for good results? This may not be an easy find, but if the tinnitus is bad enough, it may be worth the search.

In closing, here are some common questions about tinnitus.

My hearing loss is so bad that hearing aids don't help. Can I wear a masker?

If you can't hear through the aids, you won't hear a masker. But many people have reported reduction or absence of tinnitus after a cochlear implant, which is explained elsewhere in this book.

I have annoying tinnitus, but even worse is my inability to tolerate even moderately loud sounds. Are they connected?

Hyperacusis, or the inability to tolerate even sound levels of daily life, is commonly associated with tinnitus but usually involves little or no measurable hearing loss. There are varying levels of this problem, but severe cases are relatively rare. Even a mild case can cause people to want to wear ear plugs for much of their day. The volume of the world is turned to full on. It's like living in a movie with the sound track turned all the way up. This dramatically affects lifestyle for social, vocational and recreational activities. Places that provide help for tinnitus also provide help for hyperacusis. Check out: American Hyperacusis Association, 545 NE 47th St, Suite 212, Portland, OR 97213, www.hyperacusis.com

Is there any way for my family to understand what I am going through with my tinnitus?

Like pain, tinnitus is a personal experience that can't be adequately explained to someone else. However, going to a support group and allowing your family to hear the discussion may help. There is also an audio tape available called "the world of constant noise", a presentation of the maddening world of tinnitus and hyperacusis. It is 7 minutes of real life situations that occur in an average day. The Deats Scott Foundation, P.O. Box 162, Iselin, NJ 08830 (@$13)

My physician is less than helpful when I mention tinnitus, and I am not near a support group. Is there somewhere else I can get answers?

Dr. Jack Vernon is one of the leading experts in the area of tinnitus and he volunteers his time to answer questions for free! You can call him at 503-494-2187 on any Wednesday from 9:30–12:00 and 1:30–4:30 Pacific Standard Time or mail questions to him: Tinnitus Today at the American Tinnitus Association (see address above).

{ 12 }
A Proram for Better Communication

The term *redundant* came into popular usage during the development of the space program; spacecraft carried two or three redundant, or backup, systems. The reason, of course, was that an astronaut circling the moon couldn't very well send to the hardware store for a spare part; extras had to be built into the system.

Nature had the same idea in mind when she designed our method of communication. Every message we receive is redundant in the sense that it is presented simultaneously in several different ways: we get some messages through hearing, others through sight, and some make sense to us because of our past experience with language and life.

Here's an example of how hearing, sight, and life-experience interact to present a message in several different ways—all at the same time:

A small boy is playing with a plug in an electrical wall outlet. His mother rushes in and sharply yells "no!" The child gets the message, but in more ways than you might suspect.

1. The child hears the word "no," and even if he doesn't at first remember what it means, he senses that his mother is unhappy because of her tone of voice.

2. The child *sees* that his mother is rushing toward him. Her arms are outstretched, and she generally looks

quite excited and unhappy. He also sees her rounded lips, which give a clue to the fact that she's just spoken the word "no."

3. The child *knows* from past life experience—even what little he's had—that something unpleasant usually happens when his mother looks and sounds like this. He may also have a pretty good idea by now of what the word "no" means.

What does this have to do with coping with a hearing loss? Well, it shows how many different clues are available to help us figure out communication. People with normal hearing, however, usually use only a few of these clues. They must be taught to utilize the rest if a hearing loss blocks out their usual sound clues. The most important aspect of a program for better communication is the realization that *you do not need to hear each and every individual sound or word to understand speech.* You can use your remaining hearing, your eyesight, and your life experience (including knowledge of the language) to communicate more effectively.

The first part of this chapter will spell out methods to use hearing, seeing, and life experience to full advantage. The culmination of smoothly blending these talents is called speechreading—the ability to use hearing, sight, and mental processes to figure out what is being said without complete information. Exercises in speechreading will be presented later in the chapter. First, let's concentrate on some hints to improve the three major methods of communication.

Hearing

As discussed before, listening is an active (rather than passive) activity for someone with a hearing loss. Someone with normal hearing actually has to make an effort to tune out unwanted speech; you, on the other

hand, must make an effort to tune *in* to things you want
to hear.

The most effective strategy for improving hearing
skills involves avoiding or modifying situations that will
make listening difficult. The most troubling of these situations is background noise. There are two reasons for
this. First of all, an impaired hearing mechanism is
excessively bothered by background noise. Secondly,
the people around you aren't necessarily, aware of this.
People with normal hearing will usually understand that
you will have trouble hearing if they speak in an excessively quiet voice. But these same people may take you
to a noisy restaurant and have no idea why you are having trouble understanding the conversation. What
seems like quiet babble to them is—to you—a terribly
distracting commotion.

The easiest way to deal with background noise is to
change the situation or choose your location carefully.
In a restaurant, ask for a table away from the band, the
kitchen, or any other noisy spot. At home, do the obvious (but often overlooked) thing: turn off the television
or radio when you have a guest or a family chat. This
will make listening to conversation much easier.

Another hint for easier listening during background
noise is to decide what you want to listen to. It's a natural tendency to want to hear everything that's going
on, but someone with a hearing loss must make an effort
to follow just one conversation. Before you enter a difficult listening situation, make a conscious effort to
decide what and whom you plan to listen to. (Even a person with excellent hearing can't actually listen to two
conversations at once, and will switch back and forth
between the two conversations to pick up the gist of
what's being said. But this will be practically impossible
for someone with a hearing loss.) Make up your mind
and say to yourself: "While I'm here I will listen only to

Tom, and not to the conversation going on over in the corner." Once you have decided, then relax as much as possible so that stress does not interfere. Tell the person you are with that you have trouble understanding in noise, so you are not preoccupied with their reaction to your efforts at hearing them.

Think about the topic being discussed so you will be ready for the words and phrases to come. It is much easier to recognize words if you expect them. Ask someone to say a random word to you without using their voice and try to lipread them. Now have them say the name of a fruit the same way. It was much easier when you knew the topic and were expecting certain words.

And finally, stare at the speaker's lips. This may sound impolite, but it will make maximum use of your lipreading and it will help focus your attention.

Background noise is not the only factor that creates a difficult listening situation. You must also consider the distance and direction of sound. One simple way to make things easier at home is to rearrange your furniture so that guests or family members are nearby and facing directly toward you. In places where you don't have control of the furniture, plan your seating for minimum distance and maximum visibility. This will allow better use of your vision, too.

Seeing

As mentioned earlier, everyone lipreads to a small extent when listening conditions are difficult. Mouth movements are helpful in figuring out what's being said; so are facial expressions and body movements. Chances are, you've been ignoring most of these valuable clues for many years.

However, you frequently do read lips without realizing it; check for yourself the next time you're in background noise. If you're not staring directly at the mouth of the person you're conversing with, you should be. Doing this will help you concentrate and provide visual cues to what is being said. Since we know how to produce sounds with our own mouths, we seem to have an innate ability to recognize the mouth movements of other people, even though we have no training. Training, of course, sharpens this ability: a good lipreader can recognize more than just the most obvious mouth movements.

But even a good lipreader can't pick up everything, although there's a common myth that an accomplished lipreader can follow a conversation by sight alone. This is, in almost all cases, just impossible: Seventy percent of sounds in the English language are produced within the mouth and are visually obscure. Also, some sounds look exactly alike on the lips. An example of such *homophonous sounds*, as these are called, is *p, b,* and *m.* Without hearing (or figuring out from context) it's impossible to tell apart the words *pat, bat,* and *mat* from lip movements.

There's another limitation to lipreading: the human eye just can't work quickly enough to process speech by vision alone. The eye can only follow about eight or nine movements a second, while normal speech produces about thirteen mouth movements per second. And even if the eye could follow all these movements, there are still plenty of people who just don't move their mouths very much, or who have obscuring beards or mustaches that baffle the best lipreader.

Neighboring sounds also affect the way a sound looks on the lips. Note the shape of your mouth for the *t* in the words *too* and *tea.* There are also the obvious problems of poor lighting and excessive distance from the speaker. And sometimes there is an object between your eyes and the speaker's mouth. People talk with their hands or fingers near their mouth, with objects in their mouth, with papers in front of their mouth, etc.

The point of all this is to show you that despite popular misconceptions, lipreading is not the answer for a hearing impaired person—not the whole answer, anyway. Lipreading can provide valuable clues, but unless you supplement lipreading with other speechreading techniques, you just won't be able to follow many conversations.

To pick up visual cues as part of the total speechreading process, it's important that you be aware of five basic groups of sounds that are visible on the lips. We speak of groups, rather than individual sounds, because of those bothersome homophonous sounds that look alike. You won't be able to differentiate among sounds in a particular group just from seeing them on the lips of a speaker. But by combining the use of other visual cues (explained a bit later) with your remaining hearing, and the judgment gained through life experience, you should be able to deduce what's being said.

There are actually more than five groups of sounds, but many are extremely difficult to see, even with extensive training; however, it is very useful to know the five groups that can be read most easily on the lips. They are as follows:

1. *P, b,* and *m* are made with the lips pressed together.
2. *F* and *v* are formed by bringing the upper teeth in contact with the bottom lip. Unlike the first group of sounds, the top lip does not touch the bottom lip.
3. *Th* (either the th in thorn or therefore) is produced with the tongue slightly protruding or immediately behind the top teeth; the lips are parted.
4. *W* and *r* are not exactly alike, but in continuous speech they are difficult to tell apart. They are formed with a rounding of the lips, and with the w there is a slight protrusion of the lips.

5. *Sh* and *ch* (and the sounds j and y as in judge and yellow) are produced with a rounding and definite protrusion of the lips, with the lips opening more than for w and r.

The best way to start learning how to lipread is to watch yourself speak in a mirror. Try to identify the sounds from the five groups (which you must memorize, so that recognition of the groups and the possible sounds within the groups becomes automatic; when you reach this stage, you will be able to keep your mind on other cues).

While you're practicing in the mirror, notice how many sounds can't be seen on the lips; *k* and *g*, for example, are formed inside the mouth. The mouth and lip position for most vowels (a, e, i, o, u) is so affected by the consonants around them that recognition is difficult. Fortunately, vowels are easier to hear because they are usually spoken somewhat more loudly. After picking up a passing acquaintance with the groups, practice with a partner using normal conversation (and the exercises in this chapter). Remember, when you're practicing conversational lipreading, have your partner use phrases or at least whole words; if just sounds are mouthed, they will look different from the way they look in normal speech.

Other than learning to identify the basic groups, the only real trick to lipreading is practice and a constant awareness of visual cues. Don't forget to observe visual cues apart from speech, by the way. A shrug, for instance, can be a helpful clue to understanding "I don't know when he will be home." A hand motion can help make sense of the statement "I left my briefcase back at the office." A head nod will clarify "Yes, I did that." You will notice more and more about such mannerisms as you become aware of how they can help you understand. Indeed, you will probably be quite surprised at the amount of visual cues you overlooked when your hearing was normal.

Life Experience

Your experience, which adds up to knowledge of the language and verbal situations in general, is probably the most important tool you have in the speechreading process. Using life experience is essential because you're rarely going to be one-hundred-percent sure of what people are saying just by listening and looking. It is much easier to deduce what is being said if you have knowledge of what is *likely* to be said. For example, it will be much easier to understand "pick up a pound of ground beef" if you are discussing grocery shopping. If, perhaps, you couldn't understand the beginning sound of the word pound, it will be obvious from the content that the word is not mound or bound.

Researchers call this process—the mind filling in the blanks—*closure*. When the mind fills in the word or sound that makes sense (a pound of ground beef rather than a mound or a bound), it's called *conceptual* closure. Another way the mind fills in incomplete information is through grammatical closure. If we hear a sentence that sounds like "the boy are going to the park" we can fill in the missing *s* at the end of *boy*; even though we didn't hear it we know it must be there because of the word "are" in the sentence. If it was only one boy the sentence would be "the boy is going to the park." This is a particularly good example, because the final *s* on *boys* is a very difficult sound for someone with a hearing loss to pick up.

The point of all this is that you don't need to catch every word to understand what's being said. Your knowledge of the language and of life, coupled with effective use of your remaining hearing and eyesight, can restore much of the message missed by the ears alone. However, the biggest problem faced by most hearing impaired listeners is that they don't let the mind make effective closure; they get so hung up on trying to figure out two or three words that they forget the overall meaning of the conversation.

On the topic of overall meaning, it's important to remember that when people talk, they generally make sense. This means that if you are a secretary and your boss says what sounds like "start a new giraffe on this page," you shouldn't waste time spinning mental wheels trying to figure out why the devil a giraffe is wanted, and a new one at that. Instead, try making an educated guess as to what could have been said that sounds like giraffe. Carafe? No, nothing's been said about wine, so that doesn't make sense. Paragraph? That's more like it.

Along the same lines, you will have an easier time making sense of conversation if, as stated before, you know what to expect. Since a great deal of everyday chitchat concerns current events, a subscription to a newspaper or weekly news magazine will be helpful, especially when the conversation turns to topics that involve unfamiliar places and names.

You will generally find that any type of conversation is easier if you prepare in advance for it, even if you only have a few seconds to do so. If the topic suddenly turns to cooking, mull over some of the words you are likely to hear (recipe, ounces); if you are asking directions from a traffic cop, think in advance of difficult words you are likely to encounter (such as intersection, expressway). Then make a special effort to recognize these words in conversation.

Try some role playing with a partner. Invent situations, such as a post office, doctor's office, or voter registration office, and have your partner make up some words that would apply to each situation. Your partner should mouth the words silently, using no voice, while you try to lipread. Notice how much easier it is to figure out air mail and certified when you know the topic is the post office. Now that you see the value of knowing the topic in advance, you can pick situations and come up with words you are likely to hear.

For example, in a department store:

1. aisle
2. cash
3. display
4. hardware
5. gift-wrap
6. receipt
7. sale
8. refund
9. escalator
10. brand

Exercises like this are extremely valuable in enhancing speechreading skills. Here are some exercises that are commonly used in hearing therapy groups. They will help you to more fully understand some of the processes that happen when someone is speechreading. Once you understand these individual skills, you can practice putting them all together with connected speech. Try and make up some of your own after you finish these.

Remember that your goal is coping, not mastery. Don't be upset if you don't achieve perfect communication. That's just not possible; you cannot detect all sounds by eye.

Exercise 1: Being aware of facial expressions and gestures. Be aware that in our multicultural environment, gestures don't always mean the same thing to everyone. You could be misinterpreting. For example, the thumb and forefinger gesture for "OK" can be an obscene insult in some cultures. Try these activities to practice getting as much information as possible from facial expressions and gestures:

• Look at photographs in magazines and newspapers and guess at what might have been said by the subject of the photo. Does the subject look angry, questioning, sad? What things in his environment might give you a clue?

• Watch television with the sound off. Try to imagine—from the gestures and expressions you see—what is going on and what is being said.

Exercise 2: Picking up cues from various situations. Since speechreading is really a series of educated guesses, the more possibilities you can anticipate (things likely to be said) the better. To develop the habit of giving yourself more cues to the content of the message, stop and think for a moment before you go into a familiar situation. Try to predict the things that may be said to you. You'll have a better chance of understanding conversation when you know what to expect. Using your past experience predict what is likely to be said in the following examples (we've given a few samples; try to make up some more of your own):

Situation	What might be said
Out to dinner	How many in the party?
	Something from the bar?
	Are you ready to order?
	We have beans, carrots, and corn.
	Please pass the salt and pepper.
	I'll get the check.
At the gas station	Fill 'er up?
	Back up, please.
	Sorry, we don't take credit cards.
	Should I check under the hood?
	Your right front tire looks low.
	Sorry, we don't take American Express.
Registering at a hotel	Do you have a reservation?
	Double or twin beds?
	Sign here, please.

	The bellman will take your bags. Please pay the cashier when you leave.
At the bank	Can I help you? Is this for savings or checking? Would you sign the back of the check? Could I see some identification?
At the doctors	Have you been here before? Which doctor is your appointment with? Fill these out and bring them back. Have you been staying on your diet? Describe the pain for me. Your insurance will not pay for this.

Exercise 3: Recognizing the homophonous groups. Go back and review what the groups of sounds look like on the lips. Following are lists of identical-looking words within each group. Have a helper say one of the words to you silently. Be sure your partner uses normal lip movements; exaggerated lip movements will only prove distracting. You should try to determine what group the beginning or final sound of the word is in—the *p, b,* and *m* group; the *f* and *v* group; the *th* group; the *w* and *r* group; or the *ch* and *sh* group. *Don't try to guess the word—that's impossible, and you'll only get frustrated.* Guess the group. For example, if your partner silently says "bath" in an exercise dealing with the end of words, your response should be "the *th* group."

The only reason we are using words is that having your partner say individual sounds would be worthless, since the lip movements would be distorted. By the way, your partner should skip around among these lists; it will be a bit obvious if all the words from the *p, b,* and *m* group are said one after the other. Your partner should tell you whether the group sound you are guessing occurs at the beginning or end of the word.

Words beginning with sounds from the p, b, and m group:

BABE	MAKE	BAT	BEAT	MIKE	PIKE
MOOT	MAT	POLE	MOLE	BONE	BORE
PAT	BAKE	MORE	MUD	BUD	MEAT

Words ending with sounds from the p, b, and m group:

LAMB	SLAB	TOM	TOP	LAP	LAB
SLIM	COP	SLAP	CALM	SLIP	SLAM

Words beginning with sounds from the f and v group:

FAN	FEND	VAULT	FAT	VENT	VAN
VEST	VINE	VAT	FINE	FAULT	FILL

Words ending with sounds from the f and v group:

LEAF	STRIFE	STRIVE	LIVE
LEAVE	SAFE	LIFE	SAVE

Words beginning with sounds from the th group:

THIS	THAT	THROW	THINK
THORN	THERE	THOUGH	THREE

Words ending with sounds from the th group:

BATH	FORTH	PATH	MATH
BOOTH	LATH	MOUTH	WREATH

Words beginning with sounds from the w and r group:

WING	WOUND	WAIT	WEAK	WAIL	RAIL
RATE	RUN	RING	ROUND	RAKE	WON

Words ending with sounds from the w and r group:

ROAR	HEAR	DOOR	VEER
SOAR	WEAR	POUR	TEAR

Word beginning with sounds from the sh and ch group:

SHOW   SHOES   SHIP   SHIN
CHIP   CHIN   CHEW   CHOOSE

Words ending with sounds from the sh and ch group:

LEASH   WISH   WHICH   MUSH
WASH   WATCH   LEACH   MUCH

Exercise 4: Guessing words. Now's your chance to guess the whole word. Below are sets of three words (note that the words are not from the same homophonous group). You choose a set of three words. Your partner will mouth one of the three words; you must select the word based on the movements you see.

PAY, WAY, THEY
BAT, THAT, CHAT
LIME, LIVE, LIAR
RAIL, BAIL, FAIL
BOAT, VOTE, WROTE
POUND, ROUND, FOUND
MEAT, WHEAT, CHEAT
FINE, WINE, MINE
BOO, FEW, SHOE
FAULT, VAULT, MALT
THINK, WINK, MINK
CHIN, THIN, FIN

Exercise 5: Guessing groups in a sentence. Have your partner read each of the sentences silently, mouthing the words. You are to guess which group of sounds appears most frequently. Do not try to guess the sentence itself.

BOB BROKE THE BOY'S BIKE.
SHE CHOSE TO SHOW HER SHOES.
THEY RODE ROUND IN THE RED ROADSTER.
PUT THE PURPLE POLE ON THE PORCH.

THE VIEW FROM THE VILLAGE IS VIVID.
WILLIAM WENT TO WATERTOWN TO WEIGH HIS
WAGON.
THE FLAT TIRE WAS FINALLY FIXED ON FRIDAY.
THERE ARE THREE THOUSAND THESPIANS IN THE
THEATER.

Exercise 6: Practicing grammatical closure. Your brain fills in information without any conscious effort on your part. Once you've learned a language, you apply the rules of grammar even when the message is said or heard incorrectly. Have your partner read the following sentences aloud without saying the parts in parentheses. The sentences have intentional errors. The errors duplicate what people with a hearing loss might *think* they hear. Note how your knowledge of grammar enables you to correct the error without even thinking about it.

THE BOY(S) ARE GOING TO THE STORE.
THE MAN BOUGHT (A) CAR.
THAT IS SALLY('S) DRESS.
WHO (IS) COMING HOME?
HE IS GO(ING) TO THE BANK.
GIVE THE BALL (TO) JACK.
I LEFT MY KEYS (IN) MY CAR.
HE GO(ES) BACK HOME EVERYDAY.

Exercise 7: Practicing conceptual closure and flexibility. Your past experience with language and with life helps you to figure out what was said by:

a. helping you judge what might have been said, even if you didn't hear the whole message correctly
b. enabling you to eliminate choices that just don't make sense

However, in order to figure out what might have

been said, you must remain open to many different kinds of possibilities—as long as they make sense. In the sentences below, fill in the blank in at least four different ways. Be flexible, and consider all the different possibilities; remember that there are many different shades of meaning in the English language. Some possible ways the sentence can be completed are given at the end of the exercise. See if you can come up with an equally wide range of possibilities.

    a. I HAVE A BLUE_____.
    b. I WENT TO_____ON MY VACATION.
    c. I DRIVE A_____.
    d. I LIKE_____SANDWICHES.
    e. GET SOME_____AT THE GROCERY
       STORE.
    f. I FEEL_____.
    g. WHERE ARE YOU_____?
    h. THE BIRDS WERE_____.

Possible ways to complete the sentences:

    a. sweater, car, rug, book
    b. Europe, Chicago, bed, camp
    c. car, motorcycle, Ford, hard bargain.
    d. ham, huge, fresh, club
    e. milk, meat, lettuce, change
    f. sad, lonely, soft, carefully
    g. going, driving, at, looking
    h. flying, eating, beautiful, singing

Exercise 8: Practicing flexibility and homophonous groups. Now, here's a chance to combine some skills. Following are some sentences that don't make sense, but let's pretend this is the way you heard them. For each one, first decide why it doesn't make sense. Then replace one of the words in the sentence with one that would look like it on the lips (same homophonous group) but will be more sensible. The correct replacement words are shown at the end of the exercise.

    a. DID YOU TAKE A MATH?
    b. THAT MAN IS VAT.
    c. I LOST MY CHEW.
    d. I DON'T LIKE TO RATE.
    e. SHOP THE ONIONS INTO PIECES.
    f. THE TRAIN CAME OFF THE WAIL.
    g. SOMEONE CALLED A COB.
    h. SIT ON HIS LAB.
    i. WE HAD A VINE TIME.
    j. THAT WAS VERY LEAN BEAT.
    k. I'VE HAD TOO MUSH OF IT.
    l. SHE IS REALLY GETTING SLIP.
    m. THE BIRD HURT HIS RING.
    n. THE DOG SHOULD BE ON A LEECH.
    o. PUT THE SOUP IN THE POLE.

Replacement words:

a. bath	e. chop	i. Fine	m. wing
b. fat	f. rail	j. meat	n. leash
c. shoe	g. cop	k. much	o. bowl
d. wait	h. lap	l. slim	

Exercise 9: Practicing association. Fortunately, most people carry on a conversation so that the same topic is maintained for a period of time. Once you know the topic, using your past experiences you can predict what ideas and words might appear later in the conversation. Again, once you expect something, it is easier to figure out. A change in topic, of course, may throw you. Possibly you can prearrange a signal with a close companion. If the companion is talking he or she can verbally alert you to a topic change, such as "On another topic…" If a third person is talking, the companion can use a signal such as touching you in a certain way to indicate a topic change.

Given the following topics, think of at least ten words or ideas that might also be heard in the conversation. Don't be rigid—think of varied possibilities as shown in the lists at the end of the exercise.

a. BASEBALL   c. GARDEN   e. ILLNESS
b. FOOD   d. INFLATION

Words that might be heard:

a. bat, score, little league, stadium, run, hot dogs, beer, Yankees, strike, TV
b. dessert, diet, store, refrigerator, recipe, roast beef, cost, cook, splurge, cookbook
c. plant, rain, weeds, rototiller, flowers, fertilizer, seeds, rake, vegetables, bees
d. interest, banks, bills, Congress, prices, social security, economy, stock market
e. arthritis, medicine, hospital, bed, bills, doctors, pain, aspirin, fever, heart

Exercise 10: Understanding key words. Remember that because of your hearing loss and the limitations of lipreading, it is impossible to perceive every single sound or word in a conversation. But also remember that it isn't necessary to get everything to figure out the meaning of the message. You are looking for ideas, not words. If you try to see/hear every word you will be hopelessly lost, because while you are trying to figure out some words the speaker will get ahead of you. You are not required in conversation to repeat exactly what is said; you only need to react to ideas. Ideas can be communicated with just a few key words in a sentence. So concentrate on following ideas, not words. Once you have gotten a few key words, you can figure out the rest. Pick out the three or four key words in each of the following sentences. The answers are given at the end of the exercise.

a. John caught the thief yesterday.
b. The little boy cried because he lost his cat.
c. The fast car hit the truck.
d. Her cat chased the grey squirrel.
e. The girl opened the door slowly.

Key Words:

a. John, caught, thief
b. boy, cried, lost, cat
c. car, hit, truck
d. cat, chased, squirrel
e. girl, opened, door

Exercise 11: Using key words. Now, you can practice what you must do with the key words. Let's pretend that you only heard the following key words. For each item, give at least one—or maybe two—possible sentences that could include the key words. In conversation you would know which sentence is correct based on the context. Some possible sentences are given at the end of the exercise.

a. ANN	BAKED	APPLE	PIE
b. JOHN	STORE	YESTERDAY	
c. BOOK	ON	FLOOR	
d. PUT	FLOWERS	VASE	
e. BOOKSHELF	OVER		
f. YOU	READ	PAPER	
g. WHAT	ON	TV	
h. TURN	LIGHT	OFF	
i. ANOTHER	LOG	FIRE	
j. SALLY	SWAM	LAKE	

Possible sentences:

a. Ann baked an apple pie.
b. John went to the store yesterday.
   John bought a coat at the store yesterday.

    c. The book fell on the floor.
        The book is on the floor.
    d. Put the flowers in the vase.
        Put some flowers in that vase.
    e. The bookshelf fell over.
        The bookshelf is over there.
    f. Did you read the paper?
        You read the paper every day.
    g. What's on TV tonight?
        What did you put on the TV?
    h. Please turn the light off.
        Did you turn the light off?
    i. Put another log on the fire.
        Another log fell off the fire.
    j. Sally swam across the lake.
        Sally swam in the lake.

Exercise 12: Completing related sentences. Here is a chance to practice associating words and topics. Following are pairs of sentences that might follow each other in a conversation. Complete the second sentence using the topic of the first, word association, and your past experiences. For the first item one way of completing the sentence is given as an example.

    a. I went to the store to get olives.
        They didn't *have any green ones*.
    b. We saw that movie last week.
        I thought it _____
    c. Who did you vote for?
        I decided not to _____
    d. The recipe calls for two tablespoons of corn-
        starch.
        I had to use _____
    e. The flowers were wilted.
        The weather _____

Exercise 13: Forming related sentences. This time give an entire sentence that might follow the first one in conversation based on the first sentence's topic. The first item is completed as an example.

    a. Did you read the paper this morning?
       (The president's speech was in it.)
    b. TV shows are getting poorer every year.
    c. The car squealed its tires on the corner.
    d. I left those cookies on the table.
    e. The library books are three days overdue.

Exercise 14: Speechreading related sentences. Find your partner again and practice a lot of these skills together. Following are more related sentences. Your partner should read the first one aloud and then only mouth silently the second one. Using your skills of association, watching the lips, and filling in (closure), try to get the general meaning of the second sentence. Remind your partner to use natural gestures and facial expressions.

    a. The paperboy is here.
       Do you have any money?
    b. It's cold in here.
       Please shut the window.
    c. We're having potatoes for dinner.
       Do you want them mashed or boiled?
    d. It's a beautiful day today.
       I made a picnic for lunch.
    e. My car wouldn't start today.
       The battery must be weak.
    f. My social security check came.
       I'm going to the bank.
    g. Is there anything good on TV?
       I like soap operas.
    h. Would you like a snack?
       I have some popcorn.

   i. I'm having tuna fish for lunch.
     I always eat fish on Fridays.
   j. I'm working in the garden.
     I love to plant flowers.

Exercise #15: Tracking. You'll need a partner to practice "tracking", which requires you to understand segments of speech, before proceeding to the next segment. You are tracking your partner's speech a phrase at a time while you practice speechreading and your partner practices repair strategies (Chap. 5). Your partner selects a reading passage of interest and tells you the general topic. Now using a soft voice, normal lip movements, and possibly adding background noise, your partner reads the first sentence (or phrase if the sentence is very long). You repeat whatever you heard, making good guesses. If you missed any part of the sentence, your partner repeats it. If that doesn't help, have your partner rephrase, emphasize the parts you missed, give you key words, spell or write down words as last resort. Once you have it correct, your partner repeats that sentence and the next one. Continue until the whole paragraph is understood. Be careful not to get in the habit of mouthing your partner's words immediately after they are said. That is annoying to others.

Make this fun! Don't drag it out until it is a chore. Do short sessions when convenient. You can practice this yourself by using books on tape (unabridged) or tapes developed for "English as a second language" learners. Listen to the tape and then check the written text for confirmation of what you heard. Of course this will be tougher as you have no visual facial cues and there is no feedback from a partner.

Exercise 16: Listening practice. You need to practice listening with your new hearing aids. There are some sounds that will probably be very difficult for you.

Following are some pairs of words that sound similar. Sit next to your partner and hold the book in front of both of you so you can see the words, but so that you can't see your partner's face. Listen as one of each pair of words is read aloud to you. Try to determine which one was said. If you make an error, try saying both words to yourself and having your partner repeat both words several times so you can hear the difference. Practice a lot.

FEW, CHEW	SHOW, FOE
FIN, CHIN	SHORE, FOUR
FILED, CHILD	SHADE, FADE
FOUR, CHORE	LEASH, LEAF
FIT, KIT	ICE, EYES
FOUR, CORE	BUS, BUZZ
FIND, KIND	LICE, LIES
LAUGH, LACK	SEAL, ZEAL
LEASE, LEASH	FIVE, FIFE
SEW, SHOW	VASE, FACE
SIGH, SHY	LEAVE, LEAF
SAVE, SHAVE	VIEW, FEW
TAIL, PAIL	FINE, FEW
CAT, CAP	FLAT, SLAT
CUT, CUP	CUFF, CUSS
TOLL, POLE	NICE, KNIFE
THIN, FIN	TIE, THIGH
THIRST, FIRST	TIN, THIN
THREE, FREE	MIT, MYTH
THOUGHT, FOUGHT	PAT, PATH
KICK, TICK	PIKE, PIPE
KITE, TIGHT	CAT, PAT
CODE, TOAD	CRY, PRY
PARK, PART	COAL, POLE
THUMB, SUM	THAN, VAN
PATH, PASS	THAT, VAT
THING, SING	THINE, VINE

These exercises, and ones you might invent later on, will be extremely helpful in improving communication skills. However, it's also important to learn how to pinpoint the cause of a problem.

One of the most productive self-help activities for occasions when you're having trouble hearing is *to analyze exactly where the problem lies*. A breakdown in communication can't always be blamed on your hearing loss alone.

Figure 12.1 shows a model of how communication occurs; this will help you locate where the breakdown happens—so that you can decide on a method of helping yourself.

First, let's look at what could be wrong with the *speaker* and what to do about it. There are some people who speak very softly or very rapidly. They may also look down or away from you while speaking. Others mumble or don't speak clearly. The solution with a speaker problem is to let these people know that there is a problem. Be polite; take some of the blame on yourself.

"Excuse me," you might say, "I don't hear that well. Could you speak a little louder (more slowly, etc.)?" Most people are quite willing to help, but they might have to be reminded after awhile. Remember that you are asking them to change their habitual speaking habits. Try to be as patient with them as you want them to be with you when you don't hear well.

Other problems involve people with a foreign accent. You can't ask them to get rid of that, but be aware that your problem in understanding isn't all your fault.

The message that you are listening to may be the problem. If a message is long, uninteresting, or complex, it will be much more difficult to hear and understand. There isn't much you can do here, except to choose your conversations carefully. However, it does help to know why you have trouble following one conversation and not another. You can try to head off the problem with some messages by preparing in advance. If, for example, the message is a lecture, sermon, or similar presentation, find out the topic ahead of time and bone up on the subject.

The environment is an area where you have a great deal of potential for change. Communication breakdown can occur when you are far away from the speaker, when obstacles keep you from seeing the person's face, when the light source is behind the speaker's face and causing a shadow, when your hearing is blocked out by background noise or multiple talkers, or when there is a distorted public-address system.

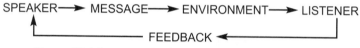

Figure 12.1 A communication model that can be used to analyze communication breakdown.

In these situations, you first have to take responsibility for your own hearing loss by making all the changes you can. Move closer to the speaker, change your position so there are no obstacles blocking your vision, turn off the radio or television in the background, or ask for a seat away from the noise. Always arrive places early so you have a choice of seats. Once you have done all you can, politely ask others for assistance. "I am having trouble hearing you. Could you move away from that light so I can see your face? (Could you take the cigar out of your mouth? Move to the next room away from the noise? Face me when you talk? Tell me when my flight is announced?)" Often, by altering the environment, you can eliminate the communication breakdown, and your hearing loss won't be so much of a handicap.

Next, let's look at the problems within you, the listener (besides the fact that you have a hearing loss). You may have an improperly functioning hearing aid, or even none at all. You could also have poor eyesight, making lipreading difficult. What about times when you are just not interested or motivated to listen and thus have poor attention or concentration on the listening task? Perhaps you have poor skills in speechreading, or are not using your knowledge to help figure out the message.

Most of these problems can be helped by a visit to an audiologist who can fix your aids or fit you with aids and give therapy for proper listening skills. However, it is up to you to check your eyesight, and to be aware when you are "tuning out" a conversation due to a lack of interest or motivation.

Videotapes can be very helpful in practicing your speechreading. Among those available are:

Lipreading Made Easy
Alexander Graham Bell Association for the Deaf
3417 Volta Place NW, Washington DC 20007
Phone: 202–337–5220
This two-hour tape, available for $75 at the time this book was written, is excellent for helping you recognize sounds.

Read My Lips
Speechreading Laboratory Inc.
4005 NW 42nd Street, Oklahoma City, OK 73112
1–800–433–6370
This series of six tapes, which costs $186, focuses more on words and sentences than the *Lipreading Made Easy* tape.

I See What You Say
By M. Kleeman ($50 for video and manual)
A self help speechreading program with multiple practice activities. Available through the Self Help for the Hard of Hearing (SHHH) catalog.

Two particularly useful books:

Speechreading: A Way to Improve Understanding, by Harriet Kaplan, Scott Bally and Carol Garretson, available for $14.95 from the Gallaudet University Press. Write to the press at 800 Florida Ave., NE, Washington, DC 20002.

What People Say, the Nitchie School Basic Course in Lipreading, by Kathryn Ordman and Mary Ralli, available for $10.95. This is a bit dated, but has some great practice materials. Write the Alexander Graham Bell Association for the Deaf, 3417 Volta Place, NW, Washington, DC 20007.

It's worthwhile to review two problems that need particular attention when designing a program of better communication: Learning to listen with one ear and coping with high-frequency (high pitched) losses.

Hearing Loss In One Ear

Often, some counseling and practice can help those with unilateral hearing losses do quite well. If they know what the problem is, they can make a conscious decision to do something about it, including developing speechreading skills, rearranging furniture and seating arrangements, avoiding noisy situations, and being assertive. Sometimes, an assistive device will help considerably.

One option is to utilize a hearing aid that routes sound from the side of the head with the non-functioning ear, to the good ear. The CROS (contralateral routing of signals) aid performs this function, usually through a wire connecting two BTE or ITE aids or through the frame of a pair of eyeglasses. If you don't wear glasses and don't want a wire across the back of your head, you can purchase an aid that transfers the sound via radio waves. This type of setup is expensive—up to $1,500— and sometimes malfunctions, but can offer convenience. A CROS system eliminates having a "bad side" for listening and sometimes helps determine where the sound is coming from. A variation of this for those with very severe loss in one ear, is an ITC or CIC hearing aid in that ear that picks up the sound on the bad side and transmits it to the good ear via bone conduction (i.e. vibrating the bones of the skull).

For background noise problems, it is often useful to purchase a personal FM system or a one-to-one communicator that feeds into the good ear. This will focus on the speech to be heard so that the background noise is not as distracting.

High Pitched Hearing Loss

Again, counseling and speechreading can help. Also, you may want to ask your audiologist about new advances in hearing aids that can custom-tailor the amount of amplification for certain frequencies or even transpose the information in the frequencies that you cannot hear, into those you can. Some of the assistive devices, such as a FM system or an infra red system, may also be useful.

With a long term high frequency hearing loss, your own speech may be affected because we monitor our own speech and if you can't hear high frequency sounds well, like s, sh, f, th, you may stop producing them in a sharp crisp manner. They may sound slurred or almost not there. Ask your friends and family to honestly tell you if your speech has changed. If this is a problem try to remember to enunciate well. If it doesn't improve, an audiologist or speech language pathologist (therapist) can help out. If you spend time with a spouse or friend who also has a hearing loss, this type of speech can be a real problem for them to understand.

Remember that all the aspects of this chapter—

speechreading, exercises to improve speechreading ability, and methods of analyzing communication breakdown—may be of more help to you if you use them in conjunction with assistance by professionals. The next chapter will explore how professionals can help you expand on self-help strategies. First let's consider some of the more frequently asked questions about these methods of improving communication.

Because I have trouble communicating, I sometimes feel as though people are walking all over me because I can't get my point across. Why do I feel this way?

Maybe it's because people actually are walking all over you. The world has no shortage of insensitive boors. However, you have a right to communicate, so don't be reluctant to assert yourself. Methods of improving assertiveness will be discussed in Chapter 14. Remember, too, that some of the responsibility rests on your shoulders. You have the responsibility to learn to speechread, to get hearing aids and learn how to use them, and to be willing to inform other people that you have a hearing problem. Once people are aware that you can't hear well, they are much more likely to make a special effort to communicate.

I'm afraid of making stupid mistakes in conversation. What can I do?

Relax. Admittedly that's easier said than done, but it's essential to learn to laugh at yourself. If, for example, you're at a restaurant, and make an odd mistake in conversation, two things can happen.

1. You can smile and say, "Sorry I have a little trouble hearing when there's a lot of noise in the background." Then the conversation goes on.
2. You can fume about your mistake, and make

your companion so petrified of talking to you that the conversation grinds to an immediate halt. There's another advantage to maintaining an easygoing attitude: Your mind works much more efficiently when it's not stricken with anger or panic. You will have a better chance of understanding conversation if you are able to be flexible, and allow yourself the opportunity to think calmly.

What determines who will be a good speechreader?

It's hard to predict, but generally we see that the most successful speechreaders are people who can use parts of a puzzle to figure out the whole thing (synthesis), have good visual skills, have a good knowledge of the language that they are speechreading, are motivated, have self-confidence, are flexible, and have a good sense of humor so they are willing to make mistakes.

{ 13 }
Hearing Rehabilitation and Therapy

After spending some time on the exercises in the previous chapter, you probably now realize the value of that type of activity in polishing speechreading skills. Whether it was apparent or not, each exercise gave you practice in doing the things necessary for good speechreading: recognizing groups of sounds in conversational speech, filling in the blanks when you don't have complete information, and learning to anticipate what sort of things might be said in some conversations.

But perhaps you really don't feel that you benefited from the exercises, and maybe you're right. Some people just don't do well in self-help situations; they may need extra explanation, or additional motivation, or help in avoiding bad habits. Some hearing impaired adults also don't happen to have a partner with whom they can practice.

So if you don't feel comfortable with the progress you've been making, it might be wise to investigate hearing therapy. The first step is to find a hearing therapist—an audiologist (or sometimes a speech-language pathologist) who has experience and interest in the field of aural rehabilitation. Not all audiologists and speech-language pathologists do hearing therapy, by the way. Some only do diagnostic testing, for example, or educational work with youngsters. But hearing therapists can be located by using the same guidelines used for finding an audiologist; they are outlined in Chapter 8. Colleges/universities or rehabilitation centers are your best bet.

If you can't decide whether or not to pursue a hearing therapy program, here are some points to consider:

• Exercises, such as the ones in the previous chapter, should be an ongoing process. In other words, you can't benefit by doing the same exercise forever. Some people have no trouble coming up with new exercises, but others just aren't that creative. A therapist, though, will have an extensive supply of exercise material.

• Working on your own may be very productive, but there's always the chance that you will get something wrong and practice a bad habit. A therapist is trained to recognize a bad habit and help you alter it before it becomes ingrained.

• There are some communication skills that are impossible to present in a book and practice at home (listening practice in controlled background noise, for example). A therapist will have equipment and materials to help you practice these skills.

• A hearing therapist is trained in counseling, and can help you deal with emotional problems. The therapist will also help with problems related to your hearing aids.

• If you go to group therapy, which is cheaper and often felt to be more effective, you will meet many people who share your problem. This will often prove to be very helpful, because you can learn a lot from the experience of others.

The choice, though, is yours. You may make perfectly good progress on your own; but on the other hand, you may become stalled, and require some external motivation to keep making progress. This chapter should, at the very least, give you some idea of what hearing therapy programs are like, and what to expect from them.

What goes on in hearing therapy? Well, a typical session lasts from one to two hours, and usually takes place once a week. Sometimes, a client meets alone with the therapist, but more often the sessions involve a group of four to ten. Group sessions are most common at colleges and rehabilitation centers; these are the first places you might consider looking for a group. Hearing therapy is typically not a long-term affair, and the group will probably meet for only four to ten weeks.

The content and style of group sessions vary quite a bit, naturally. Some sessions are highly mechanical, focusing almost entirely on lip movements. If the sessions are going to deal only with lipreading, consider passing them by. They are likely to be quite boring, and of limited value. You will benefit most from sessions where a wider group of techniques (including closure and assertive communication, for example) are taught.

Counseling is an important part of hearing therapy, too. Although counseling cannot completely take the place of training in communication skills, learning to deal with emotional problems is vitally important. The best kind of hearing therapy involves a little of everything: practice in reading expressions, closure, lipreading, advice in dealing with emotional problems, and so forth. The goal of hearing therapy should be to mesh all these aspects.

If you do decide to join a hearing therapy group (using the above suggestions to find one that's right for you) here are some ways to insure that you get the most from your sessions:
  • Make it a point to interact with the other people in your group. Learning from others is valuable.

Your sessions will also become more productive after you make friends with the other participants and become more comfortable with them.

• Feel free to offer suggestions to the therapist, who is probably quite interested in how you feel the sessions could be improved. In fact, it's not uncommon for therapists to conduct a poll of their clients, seeking their reactions and suggestions.

• If you have trouble hearing the therapist, say so. No one will be offended. If you have a very severe hearing loss and experience a great deal of difficulty in group situations, maybe you would be better off in individual therapy.

• Planning on buying hearing aids in the near future? It might be best to purchase them before you start therapy. You can still attend most therapy sessions if you don't yet have aids, but since some of the therapy will involve learning to use the aids, your time will obviously be better spent if you have them. But if you can't afford aids right now, or have some other compelling reason why you can't get them, don't automatically pass therapy by, you can still benefit.

How much should you expect to pay for hearing therapy? Prices vary quite a bit, but in most cases, you must plan on spending at least $35 to $45 per hour for individual therapy. In group sessions the cost is often split among the members; sometimes, a flat fee is charged to each member of the group. Look around. Many training institutions offer these services free or for a minimal fee.

You'll have to decide for yourself if therapy is worth that much to you. To help you in your decision, here are three case histories. Remember that these are the best of the best examples, and not everyone can make the same kind of progress. However, these case histories do illustrate the way therapy sessions deal with emotional, social, and vocational problems.

Case History 1: An Emotional Problem

Andy was very depressed about his hearing loss, and suffered from all the typical emotional difficulties: a feeling of isolation, a suspicion that people were persecuting him, and a generally pessimistic attitude toward life. Andy's wife eventually convinced him that group hearing therapy might be a good idea. The turning point for Andy came when he realized that all the people in the session had gone through the same kind of problems. Once he knew that he wasn't alone, it was easier for Andy to make a positive effort to break the depression cycle.

Case History 2: A Social Problem

Anna's hearing loss progressed to the point where she was having difficulty understanding people in group situations. As a result of this frustration, she quit all of her clubs, and she and her husband stayed home all the time. To make matters worse, Anna let her husband take over all the communication chores, such as answering the telephone and doorbell, talking to friends, and doing household business. Eventually, she got sick of this situation and decided to join a hearing therapy group offered at the local university. After a few sessions, Anna began to realize that the answer was not giving up her social life, but altering it. Acting on suggestions from her therapist and other people in the group, Anna decided to:

- Go to quiet meetings, sit close to the front of the room, and tell the people running the meeting that she doesn't hear well and would appreciate it if they spoke up.
- Get some assistive devices to help her hear in meetings.

• Concentrate on speechreading to help her understand more in noisy places.

Once she knew how to modify the things in life that gave her trouble, Anna found that she was once again enjoying herself. What happened recently is a good example of how she's learned to cope: A business acquaintance of her husband's wanted to get a few people together for dinner at a local restaurant. Instead of going to the noisy restaurant (it had a band) and straining all night to pick up threads of the conversation, Anna asked if it was all right to have a quiet dinner at her home, instead. No one objected, of course, and Anna had a fine time.

Case History 3: A Vocational Problem

Fay, a receptionist, was having a terrible time hearing people talk to her, especially over the telephone. Even though she was only fifty-six, Fay decided that it was time to retire. But retirement didn't turn out to be what she expected. Fay rapidly grew bored, and the loss of income really hurt. Finally, motivated more out of boredom than anything else, Fay joined a hearing therapy group she'd heard about. To her surprise, Fay found that over half the participants in the group still worked, many of them in jobs much like her own. Her therapist felt there were many jobs Fay could undertake, and referred her to the state vocational rehabilitation service. That agency helped her pay for hearing aids (more information on vocational rehabilitation in the chapter on money problems) and also helped her get a job at a quieter office, where she would have the use of an amplified telephone. Fay is back at work and making money, and her newly acquired communication skills are enabling her to interact with people more frequently and effectively.

Once again, these case histories are among the

most positive outcomes of thousands of cases. But good things do happen—if you make the initial effort. Whether you rely entirely on self-help material from this book or join a group, the important thing is that you recognize the need for change and take action.

The next chapter will deal with ways to take what you've learned and apply it to the real world, especially in difficult situations. First, let's examine some of the most commonly asked questions about the material in this chapter.

How can I tell if the self-help program in this book isn't working for me?

First of all, there's no reason why you can't combine the material in this book with visits to group or individual therapy, unless, of course, you live in a small town, where there are no audiologists to help you. If you want to try and sharpen your communication skills on your own, give it a month or so. If you don't feel you've made adequate improvement by then, start looking for a therapist. The videotapes mentioned earlier might be another alternative.

You mentioned that colleges are a good place to look for a hearing therapy group. If I go to a college, won't I have a student therapist practicing on me?

Sometimes, but remember that a student therapist will be closely supervised by a certified audiologist, and since the work is being done for a grade, the student is likely to make every effort to do a good job. In any event, the student's supervisor— whose business it is to train others—is likely to be a top-notch audiologist who wants to make sure you are getting useful therapy sessions.

Which is better, group or individual therapy?

For most people, group therapy is probably the better alternative, at least initially. It is less expensive and puts more emphasis on social interaction—which is what it's really all about. As mentioned before, someone with a really severe hearing loss will have a tough time in group therapy; so will someone with extreme emotional problems. Individual therapy is probably better for them.

{ 14 }
Out in the World: Assertive Communication Behavior

No matter how much your communication skills improve with practice, don't forget that even the most carefully rehearsed exercise can go astray in a real world situation. The person you're speaking with may be apathetic, uneasy, or downright hostile.

When this happens, it's time to call up what may be the most valuable trait a hearing impaired person can develop. You must be assertive.

What is assertive behavior? Put simply, assertiveness is standing up for your own rights, but not stepping on other people's rights in the process. This differs from passive behavior (where you let people take advantage of you) and aggressive behavior (where you violate the rights of others).

Here's why standing up for your rights is important:
- Because you have a hearing loss, you must be more assertive than most other people simply to insure that you can communicate.
- Because of your communication problem, there will be times when others try to take advantage of you.
- You need to feel good about yourself. This won't happen if you continually are passive or aggressive.

The last point may be the most important. As we've seen, a hearing loss is tough enough on the emotions. The problem need not be compounded by a lack of self-respect brought on by passive or aggressive behavior. Two case histories help illustrate why passiveness and aggressiveness won't help your self-image.

Case History of Passive Behavior

Vera dealt with her hearing loss by nodding and smiling a lot, even though she usually didn't have the faintest idea of what was being said. Because she didn't insist on her right to communicate, Vera felt badly about herself. "I let people take advantage of me all the time," she thought. "That clerk yesterday ignored me for ten minutes, even though he knew I was waiting. If I just didn't have so much trouble hearing, I would have spoken up." This type of behavior led to even more passiveness, because every day Vera would *reinforce* her self-image by her inability to cope with everyday situations. She became trapped in a never-ending cycle.

Passive communication behaviors include:
- just nodding and smiling while pretending to hear
- avoiding eye contact so no one talks to you
- avoiding social situations all together
- staring into space and pretending you are not interested
- letting someone else be your interpreter

Case History of Aggressive Behavior

Hans always got his way—regardless of how he hurt the feelings of others. If, for example, he couldn't make out what his wife had just said, he would snap: "Why the hell can't you speak up?" Hans found that in most cases this type of behavior enabled him to get his way, but there was an unfortunate side affect. People didn't like the way he acted, and avoided him. Even his wife began to sidestep conversation as much as possible. As a result, Hans began to feel isolated and lonely. Even though he prided himself on always getting his way, Hans, eventually, was the loser.

Aggressive communication behaviors include:
- blaming others for your problem
- insisting you have no problem
- getting angry at lack of communication
- demanding help from others, not asking
- dominating the conversation so you don't have to listen

Now let's see how taking the middle ground can pay off.

Case History of Assertive Behavior
Christine, a business woman, had learned that she could usually get what she wanted by directly expressing how she feels and what she needs; in business matters she expressed herself in an *appropriate manner*. When she first noticed her hearing loss, Christine decided that coping with it would require much the same approach. She not only held a high regard for her own rights, but respected the rights of others as well. When she entered a difficult listening situation, Christine would be likely to say: "Sorry, I don't hear as well as I used to. Would you mind speaking up a bit?" By this statement, Christine indicated that although she would like the other person to speak up, she realized that the hearing loss was her problem, and she was willing to take responsibility for it. This approach didn't always work, by the way. Christine knew from long experience that some people will refuse to be helpful regardless of what approach you take. But in most cases, Christine knew that people would respect her needs if she made an effort to respect theirs. And in any event, she would always know that she had tried, and as a result, *she felt*

good about herself. Assertive communication behaviors include:
- taking responsibility for the problem
- letting others know your responsibility by a quick phrase acknowledging the loss
- asking for, not demanding, help
- telling the person exactly what you need, i.e., slow down, look at me, a little louder, move your hand away from you face, etc.
- giving feedback to show your appreciation
- being willing to remind them at the next conversation

Remember that your attitude and the way people react to you isn't based entirely on what you say. How you say it and what gestures and mannerisms you use also play a role. For example, you will frequently have to ask people to repeat things. The way in which you make the request will play an important part in determining how successful you are. Make an effort *not* to say "what?...what?...what?" It can be enormously irritating to the person you're talking with. Instead, say back to them what you've heard of the sentence so far, for instance "John took his car and went where?" Or, "You went to the restaurant and had what?" Or, "What did you say about the shelf?"

Not only is this approach more polite than "What?...what?...what?", it also shows that you are interested in what is being said and lets the speaker know how much has to be repeated. A common misunderstanding others will have about you is that you are daydreaming and not interested in following the conversation. You know that this isn't so, but it's your responsibility to make others aware of it, too.

Responsibility plays a large role in coping with hearing loss. As part of assertive behavior, you must be willing to shoulder a number of responsibilities, such as:

1. *Changing or modifying your environment whenever possible.* If your living room furniture is not arranged so that you can easily see the faces of your guests, or the light is in your eyes rather than on their faces, it is your responsibility to rearrange the furniture. It is not your guests' responsibility to go through all sorts of awkward activities so that you can see and understand them. Likewise, you are responsible for getting and learning to use a hearing aid.

2. *Changing your behavior if necessary.* Observe how you function in various situations, and work to change your behavior if it causes you difficulty. Notice how people react to you; if you want people to react differently, try to identify what it was that you said or did to cause their original reaction. If it's something that you can change and want to change, do it.

3. *Admit that you don't hear well.* Many awkward situations develop when someone refuses to admit to a hearing problem. Remember, sooner or later your hearing loss will become obvious to people around you. If you don't admit to an obvious problem you are, in effect, telling others that you are ashamed of it. If that's the case, people around you may follow your lead and feel ashamed of it, too. But if you admit the problem in the first place, and enlist the help of others, they can give you a lot of assistance without anyone being embarrassed. Also, they won't misconstrue your behavior when they know that you have a hearing loss. They'll know that you're not a snob, that you're not stupid, and that you're not trying to hide something.

By meeting these responsibilities head on, many situations that are currently awkward for you may become easier to deal with. For example, dealing with bank tellers and store clerks can be made easier if you take the responsibility to tell them you are having trouble hearing, and then tell them what they can to do help. Someone whose job it is to communicate will usually be very receptive to suggestions on how to make things go better ("Could you speak more slowly, please, and face me?").

Although many hearing impaired people report problems with bank tellers and store clerks, using the telephone seems to be the most vexing problem. It is your responsibility to do everything you can to modify your environment and make telephone usage easier (such as getting an amplified telephone or a T-switch on your hearing aid). But after doing your part, it's not out of line to ask others for help.

The easiest way for someone to help you understand telephone conversation is to spell out the word you are having trouble with. (Remember, problems in communication often develop because of just one or two words you can't understand. Once those words are cleared up, the conversation can move along.)

Will the person on the other end of the line think it strange that you've asked him to spell out a word? Not very likely; everyone occasionally has trouble understanding over the telephone because of the instrument's inherently poor transmission. If you walk into a police station, where critical information is constantly being taken over the phone, you'll find that everyone asks for words to be spelled out. "That's May Street, M-A-Y?" "The victim's name is spelled with a C like in Charlie, A like in Adam . . . ?"

If you have really severe difficulty using the phone, it might be wise to set up this simple, proven system with friends and family: Repeat each word. If you are talking to your son, for example, he might be able to help you understand by saying, "I-I, won't-won't, be-be, home-home, until-until, six-six." Military radio operators use this method; they ask for "words twice" when reception becomes poor.

Many *hearing impaired* people have particular difficulty using the phone in an office or shop, where background noise is often very troublesome. In some cases, you should ask your employer for an amplified telephone. At the very least, try to get people in your work area to recognize your need for relative quiet when taking a phone call.

Problems in the workplace won't end with the telephone. Because of the high level of background noise, it may be tough to understand conversation. There's not always much you can do about this (you can't very well ask people to stop work altogether) but if you ask co-workers for some help you will probably get it. Remember that the Americans with Disabilities Act requires that your employer make the workplace communicatively accessible.

Following is a guide to dealing with hearing loss in the workplace. You may wish to clip these pages and keep them in your desk or locker; they contain some specific hints that we hope will be valuable. You might even wish to show this section to your employer or co-workers. First, let's list some of the most common problems encountered in the workplace. Then we'll list some possible solutions.

Common Problems in the Workplace

Background noise can be very bothersome, as mentioned earlier.

Multiple talkers are often encountered in a work area.

Talking on the telephone is difficult for most *hearing impaired* people in any situation, but work can compound the problem because of noise in the environment and the need for greater accuracy in a business conversation (as opposed to a social telephone conversation).

Talking through windows (such as in a bank) or across desks makes communication difficult for people with hearing impairments.

Using earplugs or hard hats can be difficult with hearing aids. The earplug problem is obvious; a hard hat may not fit well because of a behind-the-ear aid and it may cause any aid to squeal.

Getting exact information is difficult on the phone, as mentioned, and is also a problem in face-to-face conversations. While you can afford to miss a few words in most social conversations, you must be completely accurate when taking a client's order.

Meetings pose particular difficulty because of the need to hear people all around you.

Doing things while listening is tough for people with hearing impairments. For instance, a particular task may force you to look away from the person who's speaking, and will prevent you from picking up some visual cues. It's also difficult just from the standpoint of concentration.

People not facing you causes similar problems. Often, those people will be doing things while talking.

Possible Solutions to Workplace Problems

Binaural hearing aids, as pointed out in Chapter 6, will generally improve your hearing and allow you to get more exact information. They are particularly helpful at work, where they can make multiple-speaker situations easier and help you hear from both sides in meetings.

High tech hearing aids with digital processing, or at least digital programming, including directional microphones are recommended. Your best hearing will be done with these instruments and directional mics will help in noise, but you should consider the mics that can be switched on and off as there may be advantages to hearing well from all directions at times.

Telephone amplifiers can help you hear the caller better and also help to tune out background noise.

A quiet office isn't always an option, but letting employers and co-workers know of your needs may result in some easily made changes that will help you function better in the office environment.

FM systems. If your work situation involves hearing one person at a time, and there is noise and distance between you, a wireless FM microphone and receiver may help greatly. There are excellent FM systems for small meetings where each person has a mic that feeds into your receiver.

If you have a secretary, have him/her identify the caller before you take a call. Or use an answering machine so you can prepare for the conversation ahead of time.

Install flashing lights to signal a telephone ring, someone coming in the door, or a fire.

Moving away from a source of noise may be a simple solution to some of your problems. Moving your desk away from the air conditioner, for example, might be worthwhile.

Using your hearing protection will help you maintain what hearing you have. Don't believe that "more noise can't hurt"—it can. Just let others know that you won't hear well, so 'hold the conversation'. Talk to your audiologist about compatibility of hard hats and hearing aids.

Ask co-workers to talk one at a time. This will enable you to understand better (and might help everybody get things done more efficiently, anyway).

Use a tape recorder at meetings rather than trying to take notes. You will be able to watch the speaker's face, and you will get more complete information by playing the tape back later, than you would get from notes.

Ask for preferential seating. Try to sit up front at meetings and presentations. Get there early so you have a choice.

If you do your own scheduling, try not to put several demanding communication situations all in a row. Give yourself a break within a quieter work environment.

Be assertive; you have a right to communicate.

Organize a training session for co-workers, during which you will explain how they can help you communicate. Your audiologist may be willing to conduct the training session or at least provide you with the information that should be presented. Your place of employment or the vocational rehabilitation office may be willing to pay any fee requested. At least give out printed material if the group cannot meet.

Here's an outline of what you might present during such a meeting:

Agenda: Discussion of Hearing Loss

1. The limitations of a hearing aid: It doesn't restore normal hearing.
2. The limitations of speechreading: No one can pick up all sounds from visual cues.
3. When I can and can't hear: Hearing is relatively easy in some situations, difficult in others.
4. How my co-workers can make communication easier:
   a. talking more loudly but not shouting
   b. talking at a slower pace, but not so slowly

that it's unnatural
c. facing me when they talk
d. turning off noise sources
e. speaking to me one at a time
f. coming closer to me when they talk
g. getting my attention before speaking
5. Why even mild noise makes it difficult for me to hear and understand.
6. Dialogue among co-workers about problems due to the hearing loss.

In some cases, these suggestions, coupled with effective hearing aids and therapy, may help you keep your present job. If you can't continue in your present position, you may have to retrain for another job.

State governments have agencies that can help you keep your present job or retrain for another. These are usually called vocational rehabilitation agencies; check with your local social service agency to find out more.

The process for getting help from a vocational rehabilitation agency begins with filing an application. The agency will do an evaluation of your skills and attitudes. The agency may then provide counseling, prosthetic devices (such as hearing aids), and therapy.

If officials of the vocational rehabilitation agency decide that you can not continue in your current job, they will provide training for a new job, and help in job placement. They may follow up after you have been placed in a new job, to help during the adjustment period.

We hope the above suggestions help you to cope with the particular problems encountered in the workplace. One suggestion is relevant to both social and vocational situations, so it might be worth repeating. Keep a pencil handy, along with a small pad of paper or a pocket notebook. When you get into the inevitable situation where there's a lot of background noise—and you just can't make out those one or two key words—take out your paper and pencil and ask the person with whom you are speaking to write those words down. Embarrassing? Maybe a little, at first. But ask yourself which will be more embarrassing in the long run: asking people to jot down the words you can't understand, or asking them to repeat the statement three or four times until you get the message—if you ever do? The pad and paper approach is definitely a convenience, and you can keep pads and pencils all through the house and workplace, as well as in your pocket.

Dealing with Specific Problem Situations

Following are a few other commonly encountered situations, which probably give you some problems in communication.

Going out to eat:
This is a fun way to celebrate an event, start a romantic evening, reduce stress of a work load, entertain friends, or just enjoy yourself. But a restaurant can be a frustrating, stressful, and even unpleasant place for all involved, if even one person has a hearing loss.

Problems encountered:
- Lots of background noise.
- Many people, all talking at once.
- Seating arranged so you can't see some faces, or people are far away.
- Menus in front of faces.
- Servers who speak fast or softly and sometimes are in a hurry.
- Specific information that must be heard—what are the specials?—often with foreign words.
- Poor acoustics—hard floors, big windows, dim lights.

Solutions:

• Be assertive! You are the customer who is paying for service. Letting the staff know your needs is important, especially if you go there frequently. They will want you to come back and so should cooperate. The people with you care about you or they wouldn't be with you. So give them a chance to show their caring by letting them know what you need and explain why.

• Technology! Unfortunately standard hearing aids are usually not a big help in these situations. They amplify all the noise as well as the speech, and even seem to allow you to hear the man three tables away, but not the person across the table from you. And as the noise gets louder, everything distorts. However, the new compression aids will help make the loud noise tolerable without increased distortion. The digital programming allows a better fit to your loss so the speech signal is clearer even if it is in noise, and directional microphones focus on the voice directly in front of you so you aren't eavesdropping on other tables. And of course, two hearing aids are better than one.

• And more technology. If you aren't ready for high tech aids, or if you want even better communication in this situation, try a personal FM unit. Using it with its own earphones or with a neck loop and the telecoil on your hearing aid will cut out quite a bit of background noise. If you are with one person, give the microphone to them for their lapel. With more than one, put the microphone in the center of the table or have the people pass it around as they talk. You could also use a hard wire personal listening system, which is much cheaper, but the wire could be very inconvenient.

• Choose your restaurants well. Check out the restaurants in your area, or if in a new place, don't be afraid to walk out and go to another with better conditions. Choose restaurants:
-with quiet traffic areas on roads outside
-with good lighting, carpeting, low ceilings, curtains, tablecloths
-with a leisurely unhurried atmosphere
-without background music or entertainment

• Choose your table carefully. Avoid peak hours for less noise and a better choice of table. Or call for reservations and reserve a good table. Ask or look for:
-a booth if possible
-a round table rather than an oblong one
-something away from the traffic to the kitchen/restrooms, stereo speakers, live music, air conditioning or heating units.
-a seat facing the person you will talk to the most, a seat with your back facing the wall, and not facing the glare of windows.
-any tall objects on the table that might obstruct your view.

• Be informed. Request copies of menus for restaurants that you go to frequently so you'll have the information ahead of time and can focus on communication. Look for boards where specials are listed. It will be easier when the server then reels them off to you. Read the menu carefully so you will be prepared to tell what kind of dressing you want on an included salad or the type of beverage. Educate yourself about a particular cuisine if you are going to an ethnic restaurant. Each has its own vocabulary and dishes. If all else fails, keep that paper and pencil handy. People would much rather write than keep repeating.

• Don't be pressured or intimidated by the server. Tell him/her your problem and ask for slow clear repetition or to write it down. Remember to enthusiastically thank and tip well for a good server and then ask to get that person the next time.

Places of worship:
Problems:
   • Everyone lowers their voice in reverence.
   • The clergy are far away causing difficulty in hearing and seeing lips. Also, many of them are not trained to speak well.
   • There is often noise of clothes, rustling, pages turning, children fidgiting.
   • The music/singing/chanting can be very loud.

Solutions:
   • Talk to the clergy person about getting a group FM system for the church. It is not that expensive and there are probably many others who could benefit. Be sure it comes with a compression system so the louder sounds don't hurt. You could volunteer to maintain it after training by the company who installs it.
   • Sit close to the clergy person. For some reason, even retired clergy don't want to sit in the front pews. Yet, sitting there increases the volume of the speaker, allows some lipreading, and puts the noises of the church in back of you.
   • Ask for a copy of the sermon ahead of time. With today's computer world, that should be easy.
   • Wear hearing aids with compression and direc-

tional microphones for before and after the service. If you have a telecoil on your aid, you can use the FM system with a neck loop and won't have to remove the aids.

Hospital:
Problems:
- There is equipment running nearby causing noise.
- People tend to lower their voices.
- Hearing aids whistle when a person is lying in bed.
- Staff talk to you 24 hours a day even without your hearing aids on.
- There are many staff members and some do not speak well. They are frequently doing something else while talking to you, like reading/writing in a chart, taking blood pressure, doing a physical exam. And at times they wear masks which prevent lipreading and muffle the sound.
- Visitors often sit in front of a window so you can't see their face well.
- The telephones aren't loud enough.
- Turning the television speaker loud enough for you, disturbs the whole floor.
- The intercom system from the nurses' station isn't loud enough.
- Staff often use complex explanations with technical terms so you can't "fill in" what you don't hear. They may talk to your family instead of you because you have difficulty communicating.

Solutions:
- Be assertive! You can't expect people to help when they don't know there is a problem. Let the hospital know that you have a hearing loss, what you need and why. Of course, the Americans with Disabilities Act (ADA)of 1990 and the Rehabiliation Act of 1973 cover hospitals and thus they should be

accessible to people with hearing loss. However, each person has special needs and you must ask to get services.

• If needed, ask for volume controls on telephones or for a TTY, captioned TV or headphones for the TV, hard wire or FM personal communication systems, oral or sign interpreters for conferences with professionals. Be very polite about your requests, but if they are not fulfilled in a reasonable time, mention the ADA and ask to talk to an administrator. Incidentally, the fact that you were admitted on a weekend or holiday is not an excuse for taking several days to get you the devices you need.

• SHHH has a hospital program ($80) which is a complete guide to providing services for people with hearing losses in health care settings. It includes a guidebook, a staff training video, brochures, tips for communicating cards, staff poster reminders, and stickers with the international symbol of access for hearing loss. You may want to offer the video and posters to your local hospital before needing their services. Have a packet of materials ready to go to the hospital with you. Instruct your significant other to be sure it is used.

• Talk to all the staff who come in your room about the best way to communicate with you, like "talk to me before putting on a mask," or "shine this flashlight on your face when you talk to me at night." It's not enough to say "I have a hearing loss." Be specific as to what you need each person to do and in which situations you won't be able to hear. Don't expect them to pass the information on to others. And be prepared to remind them—they have a lot of other things on their mind. Ask that a hearing impaired symbol be put on your door or bed to act as a reminder.

• If you're having surgery, be sure to talk to your surgeon and anesthesiologist about your communication needs. You may be allowed to keep your aids in during surgery. If not, have them put in a plastic ziplock bag attached to the medical records that go with you to the recovery room. You will need to hear when they try to wake you up there.

• Don't bluff! This is information critical to your health. Be sure to clearly understand instructions for tests and medications as well as your diagnosis and treatment options. Ask for it in writing. Don't allow them to talk to your family because it is too difficult for them to talk to you. You have a right to access the information firsthand.

• Routinely ask if your medications might affect your hearing. You don't need any more hearing loss.

• Some people wear a medic alert bracelet or necklace showing hearing loss in case of an emergency. Try to always bring your hearing aids in to a hospital unless they are lost or damaged in an accident. Then ask (or have your significant other ask) for a personal amplifier.

Outpatient appointments:
Problems:

• Receptionists talk to you from behind a desk or through a window, often asking questions while looking at a paper or computer screen.

• There is frequently lots of noise in the waiting room and you don't hear when your name is called.

• Physicians are often tightly scheduled and are thus in a hurry. Slowed communication can annoy them.

• Physicians and nurses talk to you while doing an exam—not always the best conditions.

- Diagnostic and treatment information is often very technical and complex.

Solutions:

- Technology! Come prepared with optimal hearing aids, and if necessary, a hard wire or FM personal listening system.
- Alert all staff that you have a hearing loss and be specific in what you need from each one of them, i.e., look at me when you talk, use this microphone please, speak a little slower, write it down please.
- Ask to be alerted visually or by touch when you are called from the waiting room.
- Don't let their hurried time schedule get you nervous. You have a right to accessible services and good communication is part of it. Be assertive—tell them why, be polite, ask don't demand.
- Don't pretend you understand or allow them to talk to significant others about your case. Insist on clear, slow, non-technical explanations. If you don't understand, stop them and tell them so.

Travel:
Problems:

- New people, different accents, critical directions.
- Noisy transportation systems, distorted public address systems.
- Unfamiliar surroundings, including hotels.
- Fatigue.

Solutions:

- Technology! Wear your optimal hearing aids. You'll need those directional microphones, compression systems and telecoils. Take your assistive devices along as well. A personal FM system will be very helpful with tour guides, or other speakers to large groups, not to mention during all those meals in restaurants.

• Always carry extra batteries. It is not always easy to get them in an unfamiliar place.

• Hotels are supposed to be accessible when you ask for services, but many are not, especially in other countries. So, if you need them, plan to take along your own portable telephone amplifier, a device that flashes when someone knocks at the door, your own wake up alarm, and maybe even an extra loud smoke alarm. Or better yet, call ahead and request these services. If they say no, go elsewhere. Even closed captions should be available. If you can't hear fire alarms without your hearing aids, ask the front desk to alert you in some other way.

• Use a hard wire or FM personal listening system in the car. The noise level and the lack of vision for lipreading make hearing aid use very limited. And don't forget a blinker buddy to alert you to a forgotten turn signal or a device to alert you to sirens outside your vehicle.

• If you stop and ask for directions, bring a map so the person can show you, as well as tell you, how to get there. Or at least give them paper and pen to write down directions. If directions must be verbal, repeat what you hear to confirm them.

• In public transportation places, like airports, don't rely on loudspeaker systems. Ask the gate staff, or the person sitting next to you, to alert you when your flight or train is boarding or there is an announcement you should know about. Watch for any visual information as well. There should be some posted nearby.

• Since airplanes are noisy places, request a seat near the front and away from engine noise. Tell the flight attendant that you may not understand announcements, so you should be alerted to any critical ones.

• Most people experience a temporary hearing loss and discomfort, even pain, from pressure changes while flying with a cold or sinus infection. Some do even without it. But if you have a hearing loss, any additional loss from flying can cause lots of communication problems.

When exposed to changes in pressure during flying, scuba diving, or even going up a hill or elevator really fast, the pressure in the air spaces in the middle ear and/or sinuses equalizes with the outside pressure, through your nose or eustachian tube which runs from the back of your mouth to your middle ears. If those passages are swelled shut or plugged from the effects of an infection, allergies, or smoking, the difference in air pressure inside your head and outside causes discomfort, then pain, and can even pull fluid into your middle ears or rupture your eardrum.

So if you must fly with congestion or if you are someone who always has problems on airplanes, take some precautions. For 1-2 days ahead, use oral decongestants and the day of the flight use nasal spray decongestants as well. Be sure to take a dose of both about one hour before you take off, and even more important about an hour before landing. For plain allergies, an antihistamine may be better. Then on the flight use an "eat, drink, and be merry" routine. The more you swallow and move your jaw, the more likely the eustachian tube will open and relieve pressure. Tell the flight attendant why you need to keep that drink and pretzels on the way down and just keep talking (or at least yawning) to someone. A more recent advance is a set of earplugs called EARPLANES, available in drug stores for four dollars. These gradually change the pressure in your ear canal so there is a less drastic effect. However, they don't help sinus pain. You can take the plugs out between ascent and descent because it is suggested that you wear your hearing aids during flight as there may be important information over the intercom, but some people find that the noise levels in the airplanes make their hearing aids uncomfortable.

• Take extra precautions when traveling. A lot of danger signals are something to be heard—sirens, horns, shouts, intruders. So be very visually alert.

Family gatherings/parties:
Problems:
- Background noise and music.
- Several people all talking at once.
- People talking while they are eating or smoking.
- Children's voices are tough to hear.
- Poor acoustics, lighting, and seating arrangements.

Solutions:
• Be assertive! You can't hide a hearing loss. Your behavior will reflect that something is different. People may think it is because you are grouchy, angry, aloof, stupid, or mentally ill. But it is probably better if you tell them the real reason—you have a hearing loss. Then you can quickly follow up with what they can do to help. They will welcome a solution since they are having communication problems on their end as well.

• Do everything you can on your own to help before asking for help. Get two quality hearing aids with directional/dual microphones, compression systems, telecoils and anything else appropriate for you. Sit where you can see the most faces and are close to the people you are talking to. Turn off or down (or ask someone else if it is OK) any extra noise like background music, a television, a dishwasher, or video games. If that can't be done, move away from the noise.

• When in a group, explain that it will be a lot easier if one person talks at a time. It will be easier for everyone.

• Try a FM personal listening system with one conversation partner. Or even get the multi-microphone system for small groups or at the table.

• When in noise, try these steps:

> • Make a conscious decision to listen to only one person and to ignore other conversations.
>
> • Focus your vision on the speaker's lips. It helps you concentrate and it helps lipreading.
>
> • Think about the topic of conversation and what words/phrases might come up.
>
> • Relax and don't try to get every word—go for the general context. Being upset makes everything harder.

• Children are tough to hear because their voices are high pitched and thus softer (except when they are screaming and distorting their voices). Also they are rarely standing still, and they talk very fast. So, explain to them that if they want you to hear, they will have to slow down and stand still. Just don't detain them for too long.

• Find someone who is willing to go to another room or a quiet corner to talk for awhile. But be polite and don't isolate them from the rest of the group for too long.

• Be prepared to tell others, and yourself, that you may have to sit this one out and just enjoy the visuals for now.

• Don't be afraid to take breaks. Listening in this situation can be very stressful and hard work. Take a short walk or even escape to the restroom for awhile.

There are some workbooks and videotapes particularly valuable for getting along out in the world.

An excellent example is a series of tapes and workbooks by Sam Trychin, a psychologist with a hearing loss, available through the Gallaudet University Bookstore, 800 Florida Ave. NE, Washington D.C. 20002 Or SHHH (see chap. 2). In fact, the SHHH publications catalog is a fantastic resource for delving deeper into almost any topic in this book. Another captioned video is "You Should Hear What You Are Missing—Coping Strategies And Assistive Listening Devices" produced by The Texas Commission For The Deaf And Hard Of Hearing. Contact: Deaf Action Center—Hard Of Hearing Program, 3115 Crestview, Dallas, TX 75235

Telephone: 214-521-0407, email: hohdac@juno.com

To summarize some assertive communication behaviors for all situations:

For Yourself
- Use hearing aids, assistive devices and eyeglasses.
- Keep informed on likely topics of conversation.
- Learn about your friends'/relatives' interests.
- Prepare for events by reading agendas, reviews, etc.
- Be honest about not hearing.
- Acknowledge fatigue & postpone conversation.
- Inform others of how they can help.
- Tell others that it is OK to let you know when you don't hear correctly.
- Give feedback to the speaker, including appreciation.
- Don't interrupt too soon, cues may come.
- Have a sense of humor when you make an error.

The Environment
- Reduce or eliminate background noise.
- Move away from background noise.

- Keep lighting on the speaker's face.
- Reduce distance between you and the speaker.
- Position yourself so the speaker's face is visible.
- Position the speaker near your better ear.
- Have one person talk at a time.
- Use microphones/amplifiers if available.
- Keep pen and paper handy to write difficult words.

The Speaker's Voice

Ask the speaker to please:
- Speak slower.
- Speak a little louder, but don't shout.
- Look at me when you speak.
- Don't cover your mouth.
- Speak as distinctly as possible.
- Hold your head still when speaking.

The Speaker's Actions

Ask the speaker to please:
- Repeat what you said.
- Rephrase what you said.
- Say that in two sentences instead of one.
- Get my attention before you speak.
- Write down what you said.
- Spell out a word.
- Give one digit of a number at a time.
- Inform me of topic changes.
- Don't chew (or smoke) when talking.
- Don't talk to me from another room.
- Tell me if I didn't hear correctly.

The next chapter will deal with another aspect of real-world problems—money. But before moving on, here are some of the most frequently asked questions about dealing with difficult people and situations.

The other day I told someone about my hearing loss and he got so embarrassed he could hardly talk. Will this happen all the time?

No. This reaction is rare, but it does happen and therefore is worth preparing for. Sometimes, people will react with embarrassment, discomfort, or outright hostility once they learn that you have a hearing problem. People who are extremely shy might be embarrassed when talking to you, but they probably act this way because they are afraid they won't be able to converse well enough to make the grade, so to speak. The same type of person might stammer at a cocktail party when he's around people he doesn't know, and is afraid of being thought a poor conversationalist. If this is the case, a friendly attitude on your part will help put him at ease.

As far as blatant hostility, remember that when someone is hostile for no good reason, it's likely that person's problem, not yours. Sometimes, people who react with hostility when you tell them about your hearing loss suspect the same problem in themselves, but are afraid to own up to it, and subconsciously try to reject their own problem by being nasty to you. To be frank, someone who displays this type of animosity—or any sort of prejudice toward you—might not be worth communicating with, anyway.

My hearing aid doesn't help at all in noisy situations. What can I do?

Hearing impaired people have damage to their system that does not allow good hearing in noise with or without a hearing aid. Regular hearing aids amplify everything, not just what you want to hear. So it may be best to turn the volume down or just to shut it off in extremely noisy situations and avoid the distraction of the aid to rely entirely on speechreading skills. But there are alternative hearing aid circuits that help in noise as discussed in Chapter 6.

A friend of mine who's had a hearing problem for years tells me she always tries to deal with male clerks and tellers because they are easier to understand than women. Do men speak better for some reason?

No, but you may hear them better. Because of the nature of sound, it is easier to understand low-pitched voices than high-pitched voices because low pitches are louder and carry better. You may, therefore, have an easier time understanding a man. Probably the hardest person for you to understand will be a child or young teenager; in addition to having higher-pitched voices than adults, they often are not particularly careful with their articulation, they are always moving around, they use slang, and they are sometimes shy so they look down while they speak.

When I am out in the world I feel so alone at times, even my friends don't understand. Is that normal?

Support groups are the answer. It helps to get together with people who are experiencing the same things you are. And your friends and family members can benefit from going with you and interacting with the significant others of the people with hearing impairments. The national Self Help For Hard Of Hearing People, Inc. (SHHH) is an excellent resource with an interesting bi-monthly magazine and a fun and informative annual convention (see address and phone number in chap.2). This group can also refer you to over 250 local SHHH groups across the country. Their monthly meetings provide wonderful support and information.

For those who are congenitally deaf, The National Association Of The Deaf is more appropriate (also see chap.2). And people who acquire deafness in later life may find support in the

Association For Late Deafened Adults (ALDA). There are even more specific support groups such as the Meniere's Network (800-545-HEAR) and the American Tinnitus Association (see Chapter 11) which can also refer you to local groups.

{ 15 }
Money Problems

When considering the cost of hearing aids, don't forget that you are paying for research and development of hearing aids, an average of five hours of service and counseling by the dispenser within the first year, and the warranty as well as the instrument itself.

There's a good possibility that you are concerned about the typical hearing aid prices that were mentioned earlier. Well, your reaction is perfectly natural. There's no question that hearing aids are expensive, and most people—when they first learn how much an aid will cost—react by asking, "Isn't there some program that will help pay for this?"

Unfortunately, these people are usually disappointed. Medicare, (medical insurance after 65 or if disabled), a federal program you've probably been paying into for quite some time, won't pay for anything to do with the eventual purchase of a hearing aid. This is unlikely to change because there are so many people over 65 who need hearing aids that mandating payment for aids could bankrupt an already shaky system. Medicare will pay for a hearing test if it is used in the diagnosis of a medical problem, but not for any testing done that is connected with a hearing aid. So be sure that any bill you or the audiologist submit for the hearing test does not mention the words "hearing aid."

Medicaid (for low income people of any age), on the other hand, may help in certain cases. The program is administered by the individual states, and varies widely among individual jurisdictions. In some states, Medicaid may provide payment for the hearing evaluation and assistance toward the purchase of an aid, along with a limited amount of follow-up care. Other states, though, provide very little.

How do you find out what your state's Medicaid system will pay for? First, look in the listing of state offices in your phone book; you will almost certainly find a listing for "social services." Call this department and ask for information about Medicaid coverage. If you don't find that listing, or a similar one, try the state's general information number, usually found at the beginning of the listings. If that doesn't help, ask your audiologist.

Don't get your hopes up about Medicaid, by the way. As noted earlier, your state may not have any benefits related to buying a hearing aid. With the current cost–cutting fervor, existing government benefits may be modified or cut back altogether. (This is why a listing of state-by-state benefits was not included in this book. These programs are currently in a state of flux, and any information gathered at the time of this writing could be inaccurate shortly after the first printing.) Also, keep in mind that you must meet certain low–income standards to qualify for Medicaid benefits, and the required investigation of your personal finances can be a demeaning process.

If you haven't yet reached retirement age, check into your state's vocational rehabilitation program (see Chapter 14). These are designed for people who are still of working age but who have lost a job or have trouble keeping a job because of a handicap. Vocational rehabilitation programs may, in some cases, help pay for hearing aids and provide counseling and job retraining. Like

Medicaid, vocational rehabilitation programs are being modified, and also vary widely from state to state. Some states even help women over age sixty-five whose job is to maintain their own home. To find out what's available in your locality, scan the state office telephone listings for any department with the word "vocational" or "rehabilitation" in the title. If this doesn't work, call the social services office, or ask your audiologist for help.

More and more private insurers are paying for at least part of hearing aids. But be aware that some will pay a specific amount (say $700) and won't let you add to it to get a more expensive aid. The majority still don't pay for the cost of aids nor learning how to use them, but it's worth it to check on yours. Call your health insurer to find out.

In a few special cases, local fraternal groups, such as the Rotary Club, Quota Club, the Lions or Kiwanis may pay for part or all of an individual's hearing aid cost. However, this is done on a case-by-case basis. If you think there is a compelling reason why one of these organizations would want to help, apply, by all means. The Sertoma Foundation is a private social service program that provides hearing aids to eligible people. For information, contact: 1912 E. Meyer Blvd. Kansas City. MO 64132-1174. Phone: 816-333-8300 Fax: 816-333-4320, infosertoma@sertoma.org. www.sertoma.org.

HEAR Now (9745 E. Hampton Ave. Ste 300, Denver, CO 80231-4923, Phone: 8000-648-4327 Fax: 303-695-7789 jostelter@aol.com, www.leisurelan.com/~hearnow/) has funds to provide hearing aids for needy people. The related services are donated by local hearing aid dispensers.

In some communities there are hearing health care professionals who volunteer their time to fit reconditioned aids at minimal costs. Or there may be loaner banks that allow you to borrow an aid for awhile until you can gather money to buy one. But remember that you will probably only get one aid from these sources and it may not be the ideal fit for you. Also, getting high technology is unlikely. Ask your audiologist or social worker about these sources.

There aren't too many other possibilities for finding money to pay for your hearing aids. But even though there is not much in the way of financial assistance, you can help yourself by shopping wisely and not spending money you don't have to. If you do end up paying the bill, don't forget that the whole cost is tax deductible as a medical expense.

Another helpful hint is to have your aids reconditioned when, after a couple of years, they develop common wear-related problems. When an aid is reconditioned, the dispenser ships it to the factory, where technicians replace most of the internal workings. Cost of reconditioning depends on the age of the aid, but on a three-year-old aid, for example, reconditioning will generally run $100-200. After reconditioning, you've essentially got a new instrument in your old case, and it may last for five more years, as long as your hearing doesn't change. Of course, if you have programmable/digital aids, a change in hearing does not require new aids.

Because a hearing aid is a substantial investment, you will want to cover the reconditioning with a one year warranty (a one year is only slightly more than a 6 months one and worth the extra money) which is about $100-200 (slightly higher for CIC or high tech).

As mentioned earlier, you can often save money on services related to hearing aids (fitting the aid, or hearing-therapy sessions, for instance) by finding a university or college-sponsored clinic in your area. Rates will probably be considerably lower than those charged in non-training facilities. You will, in most cases, be working with students; these students are under the direct supervision of a qualified audiologist. The only problem you're likely to encounter is that students need more time to conduct tests than experienced audiologists do. But if you've got the extra time to spend, the college clinic will be well worth it.

Although college audiology clinics may help with hearing tests, hearing aids, and therapy, you won't be able to avoid that required trip to the physician, as discussed in Chapter 7, nor should you try. It is essential to be sure that there's no dangerous medical problem causing your hearing loss. (It's unlikely that there is one, but you're better off playing it safe.)

A visit to the doctor should be covered by your health insurance. If the physician's appraisal is not covered by your insurer, you can save some money by scheduling the exam at a public clinic. In any event, expect a hefty fee for a visit to any specialist, especially if it's your first time at the office. Most of the time your primary care or family physician can do the exam.

Perhaps, then, you feel that this chapter has added up to a big, fat zero because it doesn't offer any magic formula for getting financial aid. Unfortunately, it is true that almost any other health problem is dealt with by more social and/or public assistance programs. However, if you add up the costs and balance them against what you are really paying for, you may not feel so bad. When you shell out something like $1,500-5,000 for a pair of hearing aids, you are actually purchasing another sense, an ability to communicate. You will use your hearing aids far more often than the family car, and will certainly get better mileage from them. On the average a pair of standard hearing aids lasts about five years which brings the cost to less than one dollar a day. Even a $5,000 pair of digital aids costs only $2.73 per day, or analog programmable aids about $1.64 per day. So stop trying to save all your money for tomorrow or for the kids. Indulge yourself—you deserve it.

Some of the money you spend for an aid also goes toward research and development by the hearing aid manufacturer, in much the same way as part of the price of gasoline pays for the oil companies' exploration for new petroleum deposits. This added cost is considerable, but judging by the recent great advances in hearing aid technology, it is well worth it.

There's also a question of supply and demand. Companies just don't sell that many hearing aids, and because few units are sold, the individual price remains high. Basically, this situation exists because only a fraction of the people who need hearing aids actually buy them. If it's any consolation, by deciding to take the plunge and buy today's relatively expensive hearing aids, you've become part of the solution to the overall money problem.

The next chapter will conclude our exploration of coping with hearing loss. First, some typical questions on money matters:

I'm pretty handy at fixing my radio. If something goes wrong with my aid, can I try and save money by fixing it myself?

A thousand times, no! Unless you are an electronic engineer with a laboratory full of equipment, you don't stand a chance of being able to fix the aid. You will only damage it further and make the repair bill even worse, and will probably also invalidate the manufacturer's warranty. Take it back to the dispenser and stick to fixing radios.

I've seen mail order ads for hearing aids. Should I consider buying one of these?

Because hearing aids are supposed to be individually prescribed to deal with specific hearing disorders, there's little chance that any instrument purchased through the mail will come close to fitting your needs. The earmold that comes with it won't be an exact fit, as would a custom-made model. Also, you won't get necessary services and adjustments when you order an aid through the mail, so what seems like a good bargain probably isn't.

I'm not sure I can come up with the money for a hearing aid all in one chunk. Can I buy one on installment?
Some hearing aid dispensers will allow you to pay over a period of time; the only way to find out is by asking. If you are expected to pay interest, ask for a clear and direct explanation of the interest rate, and be sure to find out the total amount you'll have to pay. If your loss is mild, you might start with a hearing enhancer. Resound makes one called AVANCE. This tiny BTE is hardly visible and costs under $500. However, you should go to an audiologist for a full test just to be sure that this device is appropriate for you.

As a veteran, can I get free hearing aids?
Only if your loss was service connected. But if you can pay for the aids, VA clinics are good places to get them.

{ 16 }
Coping

One thing that often puzzles doctors and audiologists is the common reaction of people who are told they have a hearing loss. "Oh God!" they say, "Do I have to wear hearing aids?"

No, of course they don't *have* to—but isn't that entirely the wrong attitude, anyway? If you feel that way...if you dread the thought of having your suspicions confirmed by a hearing test, or of wearing the hearing aids you know you need, or having to live with a permanent hearing loss, stop and think for a moment. Wouldn't it be better if you looked at it this way?

Just a few years ago, very little could be done for people with hearing losses. Today, there are concerned professionals who can help me regain a sense.

We hope that this book has given you the motivation to do something constructive about your hearing loss. We hope, too, that you will conclude that while a hearing loss means that things will change, those things don't always have to change for the worse. Coping with a hearing loss means altering your environment when and where you can. You may have to rearrange the furniture in the living room in order to see your guests' faces more clearly. Does this mean that since your living room must be different, it must be worse? No, of course not. The same type of reasoning applies to most of the new lifestyles you must adopt to deal with your hearing loss.

It's not all as simple as rearranging the furniture, of course, and you will have to live within certain limitations. But by polishing your communication skills and emotionally accepting the problem, you can keep those limitations to a minimum. There's a tendency for people with a hearing loss to let it grow all out of proportion in the total scheme of things.

Sometimes the hearing loss becomes the dominant force in their lives with every depressing minute spent thinking of how much better things would be "if only I didn't have something wrong with me."

Well, *there's nothing wrong with you*. There's something wrong with your ears, of course, but your ears are just a small part of all the things that are you. You'll have to come up with your own formula for evaluating self-worth; perhaps you value your honesty, or pride yourself on a lifetime of accomplishment and hard work. But whatever you use to gauge your self–worth, the state of your hearing should play no part in it.

In fact, there's something to be said for dealing with adversity; because of your lifetime of experience, you certainly know this. That makes you better able to cope with your hearing loss and emerge a stronger person.

Unfortunately, there are people who just don't feel up to the challenge of meeting the problem head-on. If you're tempted to take this attitude, remember that you are not the only one who will be affected. If you suffer, so do the people who love you. If you punish yourself, you punish them, too, for it will hurt them to see you depressed, isolated, and lonely.

Throughout this book, we've stressed the fact that a hearing loss is a common problem; millions of people are in the same boat as you. But don't interpret this as meaning that you should decide not to do anything about it. Bad backs are common too, but if you developed a painful back, chances are you would try to get it taken care of as quickly as possible.

Plenty of people, young and old, haven't let hearing problems slow them down: President Ronald Reagan had a hearing loss and dealt with it successfully through his terms. Others who have not let hearing loss stand in their way include actresses Nanette Fabray and Florence Henderson, actors Richard Thomas, Burt Reynolds, Lou Ferrigno, Leslie Nielsen, Richard Dysart and Eddie Albert. Comedians Bob Hope, Phyllis Diller and Norm Crosby, and sports personalities such as Bobby and Al Unser, Curtis Pride and Mike Singletary. A hearing loss didn't stop former Surgeon General C. Everett Koop, or the man often considered the greatest golfer in history, Arnold Palmer.

These people found that there was help available, and they took advantage of it. You can, too.

APPENDIX:
WORLD WIDE WEB RESOURCES FOR THE HEARING IMPAIRED

Any book published in the 21st century cannot ignore the Internet and its incredible resources on any topic, including hearing loss. Almost any search engine (a program designed to look through the Web and list web sites that match your request) will bring up thousands of references if you type in only 'hearing loss'. There are almost 10,000 related to tinnitus alone.

But this information overload can be confusing, so for those of you who don't have hours to surf, following are some web site suggestions. Keep in mind that web sites change frequently so these may not all be valid by the time you read this book. But often one of these sites can direct you to sites that did not even exist at the time this book was published. Some of the sites may seem a bit technical in places, but may have information further in that is more appropriate for you.

Keep in mind that while the Internet can put thousands of people in touch with each other and with information sources, information is transmitted over the Web regardless of whether it is true or not. Also, discussions on the Web are not monitored or edited by any authority for accuracy or attitude. Thus, your contact could be a valuable source, or a rascal out to make trouble and/or feel a misguided sense of importance.

Brand names are important. Web sites of reputable hearing care associations, government institutions, and universities usually have passed a review process. A site tends to be more legitimate if: additional sites are offered as links, information has been updated, limitations and risks of new treatments are listed and experts can be checked out through their place of employment, or credentials.

Information About Hearing And Its Disorders

www.searchwave.com—A search engine for audiology, hearing loss, hearing aids, and the ear. For practitioners and patients.

www.bcm.tmc.edu/oto/studs/midear.htm—Common diseases of the external and middle ear.

www.mayohealth.org—Mayo Clinic health oasis (search under "hearing" or "ears").

www.sinuscarecenter.com—Brochures about ears and hearing.

www.hearingbalance.com—Includes the vestibular balance system as well as hearing and tinnitus.

www.AudiologistOnLine.com—Free, live interactive consultation with audiologists. It offers a library of current hearing loss information, frequently asked questions/answers, and links to other resources.

www.healthtouch.com—Healthtouch—look under ear, nose & throat problems and hearing.

These may or may not have anything on hearing at the time you go to them: www.medscape.com and www.medicinenet.com.

www.neurophys.wisc.edu—Search for "ears"—then click "auditory animations"

Information About Hearing Rehabilitation, Services and Products

www.cochlear.com—Website of a company that makes cochlear implants and has the latest information in that area as well as links to other hearing health organization sites.

www.cochlearimplant.com—Website of another manufacturer of cochlear implants.

www.HearBetterNet.com—Shopping and information associated with American Hearing Aid Associates— nationwide network of independent hearing health care providers with products from many manufacturers.

www.hearing-loss-help-co.com—Go to captioned videos to see a list of 10,000 captioned videos which can be purchased along with other assistive devices.

www.hearingnetwork.com—Nationwide hearing health-care community and directory. Main page is designed to match consumers seeking hearing health products, services and information with their network members in their area.

www.Hearingmall.com—EAR, Inc.—national referral program for hearing health care products and services— one stop shopping.

Associations And Agencies

www.audiology.org—American Academy Of Audiology— professional organization.

www.asha.org—American Speech Language Hearing Association—professional organization.

www.ata.org—American Tinnitus Association—research and consumer support group.

www.nih.gov/nidcd—department in the National Institute

of Health that deals with deafness and other communication disorders (under health information/hearing and balance).

www.shhh.org—Self Help for the Hard of Hearing—consumer support group.

www.alda.org—Association for Late Deafened Adults—consumer support group.

www.earfoundation.org—Click on Online Support Groups

www.nih.gov/nia—National Institute on Aging.

www.aoa.dhhs.gov—Administration on Aging—opportunities and services to enrich lives of older persons and support independence.

www.audiologyawareness.com—Audiology Awareness Campaign—a not for profit foundation to educate the public about hearing losses, provide brochures, resources to find an audiologist, and a questions and answers board.

If you own a computer and are connected to the Internet, you probably also have e-mail, which in most cases is preferable to snail mail (letters through the postal service). It's much faster and you can get responses almost immediately if you are both on line. You also don't have to deal with poor handwriting.

In some cases e-mail is better than the telephone. It is less expensive, much easier to understand, you can ignore a message for days, and you have time to compose a response. You also can have a permanent copy of the "conversation" with correct spellings of names, numbers, etc. Whole texts can be sent as an attachment or "pasted" right into the e-mail message, saving lots of time. In fact, e-mail is the best thing since fax for people with hearing loss. Not too many people have fax machines out of offices, but more and more households, as well as businesses, are going on line.

Take advantage of the web sites and e-mail addresses of companies with whom you do business. It's efficient, effective, fast, dependable, and fun.

Make some contacts with other people who have hearing losses and start an on-line support group. There are already chat groups based on hearing loss. For a tinnitus chat group visit: http://chat.yahoo.com (click on: start chatting, change room, health and family, user rooms, tinnitus). Or try www.cccd.edu/faq/tinnitus.html for a lay person's response to frequently asked questions (faq's).

The Say What Club (www.saywhatclub.com) is an on line group of over 200 late-deafened, hard of hearing, and other interested folks who provide support and encouragement to each other through e-mail. This international group provides a friendly, good-humored place to exchange conversation, information, advice and chit chat.

Glossary

Air Conduction: Transmission of sound to the inner ear by way of the ear canal and the middle ear.

Anvil: The center bone of the three bones (ossicles) in the middle ear that transmit sound vibration. (Latin incus.)

ASP: Automatic signal processing—methods of altering the input to analog hearing aids to improve hearing.

Assertiveness: Behavior that allows people to request their own rights without interfering with the rights of others.

Audiologist (aud ee OL oh jist): A person who holds a degree and certification/licensing in the areas of identification and measurement of hearing impairments, and rehabilitation of persons with hearing impairments.

Auditory nerve (AUD i tor ee): The cranial nerve carrying information from the inner ear to the brain.

Aural rehabilitation (AUR al): Educational/therapeutic procedures used with hearing impaired persons to improve the effectiveness of their overall communication ability.

Binaural aids (bine AUR al): Two separate amplification systems worn simultaneously on two separate ears of the individual.

Bone conduction: Transmission of sound to the inner ear by applying vibration to the bones of the skull.

CIC: Completely-in-the-canal aid: a small amplification device, extending from 1 mm to 2mm inside the opening of the ear canal to near the eardrum.

Cerumen (sir ROO men): Wax that is produced in the ear canal.

Closed-captioned television: Printed text shown on the television screen for certain shows when an adapter is turned on.

Closure (CLOZE yure): The ability to recognize a whole, when some of the parts are missing.

Cochlea (COKE lee uh): The hearing part of the inner ear—which resembles a snail shell—and changes sound into nerve impulses.

Cochlear implant: A device that enables persons with profound hearing loss to perceive sound, consisting of an electrode array surgically implanted in the inner ear which delivers electrical signals to the eighth nerve and an external amplifier which activates the electrodes.

Communication disorders: Any interference with an individual's ability to comprehend or express ideas, experiences, knowledge, or feelings.

Conductive hearing loss: A deficit in hearing caused by an abnormality in the outer or middle ear.

Decibel: A measure of the intensity (loudness) of a sound.

Digitally programmable hearing aid: A hearing aid where the characteristics are set and adjusted using a microcomputer allowing more specific fitting and flexibility for future adjustments.

Directional/dual microphone: A microphone system that is more responsive to sounds coming from the front than from behind, and thus helps hearing in background noise.

Discrimination (acoustics): The degree to which one is able to hear and recognize differences among the speech sounds, i.e., the ability to understand speech once it is loud enough to hear.

Dispensing audiologist: An audiologist who sells and fits hearing aids, evaluates hearing, and provides some aural rehabilitation.

DSP: Digital signal processing—improving hearing with manipulation by mathematical formula of a signal that has been converted from analog to digital.

Eardrum: A thin, concave, parchment-like membrane that stretches across the ear canal and separates the outer ear from the middle ear.

Earmold: A plastic-like fitting in the outer ear, designed to transmit the amplified sound from a hearing aid into the ear.

ENT specialist: A person who holds a degree in medicine and who specializes in the treatment of problems associated with the ear, nose, and throat. Also called otolaryngologist or head and neck surgeon.

Eustachian tube (yus TASHE an): An air duct/drainage tube from the area back of the nose to the middle ear.

Feedback (acoustics): Sound that escapes from the receiver of a hearing aid or other amplification system and reaches the microphone, producing a squealing sound.

Footplate: The base of the stirrup, which rests on the oval window in the middle ear.

Frequency (acoustics): A measure related to the pitch of a sound.

Hair cells: The sensory receptors in the inner ear that translate the sound vibration into messages that go into the brain.

Hammer: The first and largest of the three bones (ossicles) in the middle ear that transmit sound vibrations. (Latin malleus.)

Hearing aid dealer: A person who sells and fits hearing aids. Many dealers prefer to be called dispensers.

Hearing aid dispenser: A person who sells and fits hearing aids.

Hearing aid evaluation: A process of determining what type of amplification system would help to utilize the patient's residual hearing.

Hearing ear dog: A dog that is trained to alert its hearing impaired master to auditory signals such as doorbells, smoke alarms, wake-up alarms, baby cries, etc.

Hearing evaluation: A measure of the capability of a person's auditory system to perceive and interpret sound. A determination of the extent and type of hearing loss.

Hearing screening: A gross measure to separate out those persons who require special help for a hearing problem.

Hearing therapist: An audiologist or speech-language pathologist who provides aural rehabilitation.

Homophonous (ho MOF en us): When two or more sounds look identical on the speaker's lips.

Impedance measurements: A physical measurement of a sound reflected off the eardrum and analyzed to reveal characteristics of the middle ear.

Inner ear: The interior section of the ear where sound vibrations and body positions (balance) are transformed into nerve impulses.

Lipreading: Getting cues from the mouth and face about what sounds were said. See speechreading.

Meniere disease (min YAIR): An over accumulation of fluid in the inner ear causing a fluctuating hearing loss, and episodes of dizziness, roaring sounds in the ear, and a feeling of fullness in the head and ears.

Middle ear: The section of the ear extending from the eardrum to the oval window.

Nerve deafness: A misleading term often used to describe a sensorineural hearing loss.

Oral interpreter: A professional who sits facing a person with a hearing loss while repeating/rephrasing what a speaker is saying using good lip/facial movements and modifying some difficult to see words.

Ossicles (OSS i culls): The tiny bones in the middle ear that transmit the sound vibrations. They are known as the hammer, anvil, and stirrup, and are listed individually in this glossary

Otitis media (oh TITE is MEE dee uh): Inflammation of the middle ear, usually caused by infection.

Otologist (oh TOL oh jist): A person who holds a medical degree and specializes in problems in the ears.

Otosclerosis: Remodeling of bone by resorption and then new formation around the stapes and oval window, resulting in stapes fixation and related conductive hearing loss.

Otoscope (OH toe scope): An instrument for visual examination of the ear canal and eardrum.

Ototoxic (oh toe TOX ic): Poisonous to the ear, usually referring to drugs.

Outer ear: The external funnel-like structure for receiving sound; it includes the pinna, the ear canal, and the eardrum.

Oval window: A membrane, the resting place of the stirrup, which pulsates with vibrations of the middle ear and transmits them into the fluid of the inner ear.

Pinna (PIN uh): The part of the ear that is visible on the outside of the head.

Presbycusis (prez–buh–CUE–sis): Hearing loss due to the aging process.

Pure tone (acoustics): A sound at only one frequency (pitch) with no harmonics.

Real ear measurements: A method of evaluating a hearing aid that takes into account the hearing aid and the specific ear by putting a tiny probe microphone near the eardrum.

Recruitment (re CROOT ment): A phenomenon sometimes accompanying a sensorineural hearing loss in which a slight increase in the intensity of a sound results in a disproportionate increase in the sensation of loudness, causing over sensitivity to loud sounds.

Resonance (REZ oh nance): The vibration of an object or a body of air where certain pitches are made louder; this is the effect noted in blowing over the top of a bottle.

Semicircular canals: Three looped bony tubes in the ear that help to maintain a sense of balance.

Sensitivity (acoustics): Ability to react to varying degrees of a stimulus such as sound; usually referring to the softest level that can be heard.

Sensorineural hearing loss (sen sor ee NOOR al): A deficit in hearing caused by an abnormality in the inner ear or the auditory nerve.

Speech pathology: Also known as speech–language pathology; the study of speech, language, and voice disorders for the purposes of diagnosis and treatment.

Speechreading: Utilization of auditory and non-auditory cues—including lipreading—to comprehend what is being spoken.

Speech recognition threshold (SRT): The softest intensity level at which one can recognize easy speech. Also called speech reception threshold.

Speech therapist: A person who has a degree and certification/license in the areas of diagnosing speech, language, and voice disorders, and of implementing therapeutic measures. Also called a speech–language pathologist.

Stirrup: The third and smallest bone (ossicle) in the middle ear that transmits sound vibrations. (Latin stapes.)

TDD: Telecommunication device for the deaf. See TTY.

Text telephone (abbreviated TT): See TTY.

Tinnitus (TIN ih tus, or ti NIGH tus): A ringing or roaring sensation in the head or ears, which usually is found with auditory impairment.

Tinnitus masker: A hearing aid–like device that produces a noise that may cover up the internal ringing, buzzing, or roaring sounds experienced by many hearing impaired people.

T-switch: An adjustment on a hearing aid that activates an inductance wire so that the aid can pick up electromagnetic waves from a telephone receiver or a group amplification system.

TTY: A telephone system for the severely hearing impaired where a typewritten message is transmitted over the telephone lines and is received as a visual message. Also called a TT or a TDD.

Tympanum: The tympanic membrane (eardrum) or cavity (middle ear).

Unilateral loss: Hearing loss in only one ear.

Vocational rehabilitation: Evaluation and retraining for employment when a disability prevents a person from doing a previous job.

Volume wheel: An adjustable device to make a sound louder or softer; often found on hearing aids or telephone receivers.

Word recognition testing: Measurement of an individual's ability to understand words once the words are loud enough.

Index